# Herbal
# Medicine

## NATURAL REMEDIES

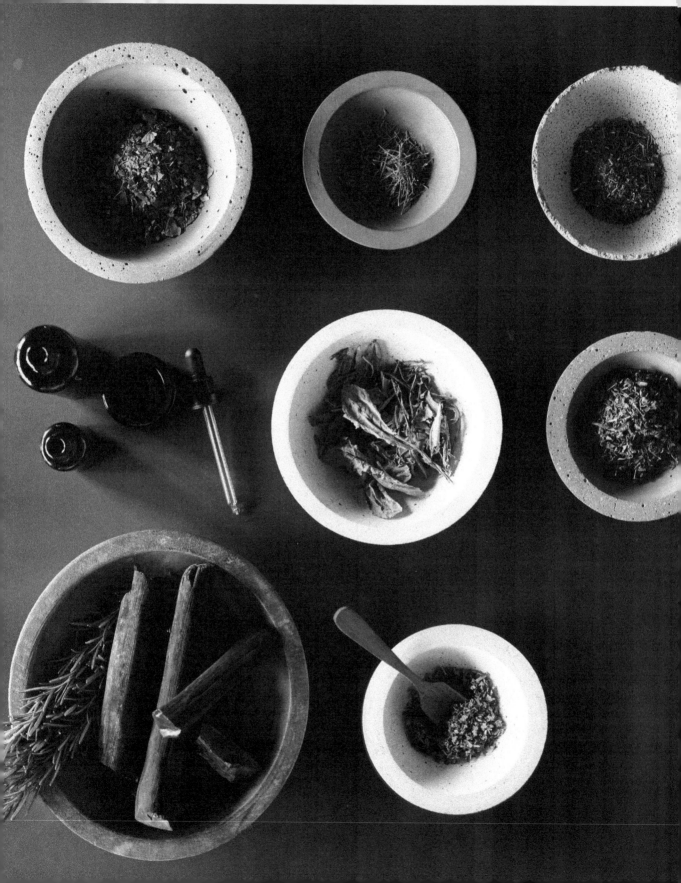

# Herbal Medicine

## NATURAL REMEDIES

## 150 Herbal Remedies to Heal Common Ailments

Anne Kennedy

ALTHEA
PRESS

For general information on our other products and services or to obtain technical support, please contact our Customer Care Department within the United States at (866) 744-2665, or outside the United States at (510) 253-0500.

Althea Press publishes its books in a variety of electronic and print formats. Some content that appears in print may not be available in electronic books, and vice versa.
Cover photography © Alicia Cho; Hélène Dujardin; Shutterstock.com; Shannon Douglas; Interior photography used under license from Stocksy/Trinette Reed, p.2; Stocksy/Vera Lair, p.8; Pixel Stories, p.18; Stocksy/Trinette Reed, p.28; Stocksy/ Alicia Bock, p.180; Stocksy/Natasa Kukic, p.222

All other images are © shutterstock

Hardcover ISBN: 978-1-63878-846-1
Paperback ISBN: 978-1-62315-852-1
eBook ISBN: 978-1-62315-853-8
R1

# Contents

# Introduction

Herbal medicine has been used for thousands of years; in fact, its history goes back much further than that of today's pharmaceuticals. It is a major component of alternative medicine, and is useful in preventing and treating a number of common ailments.

Nature's pharmacy is extensive, filled with herbs that possess powerful medicinal properties. With guidance and knowledge, everyone has the ability to use herbs to ease discomfort and promote healing.

Growing up in the mountains of Montana, I would hear stories about how Native Americans healed all kinds of illnesses using remedies made with some of the wild plants that grew just outside our family's door. It wasn't until adulthood, though, that I began to experiment with anything beyond the simplest peppermint and chamomile teas. Today I delight in growing an abundance of fragrant herbs in my garden and in the hardwood forest behind my home. I take great pleasure in walking through the woods and along riverbanks, spotting plants with medicinal properties, and marveling at their beauty

and efficacy while breathing in their fragrances. On those rare occasions when I'm not feeling well, I am often able to take care of myself by using plants I've harvested and prepared.

Some herbal remedies involve using plant parts in their fresh, natural state. Others call for store-bought extracts, and still others for compounds made in the comfort of your own kitchen. By conducting a bit of research, ensuring that a specific herb is right and safe for me, and following any applicable precautions, I've been able to easily take charge of my own health and treat minor ailments before they worsen and require medical intervention. Now you can, too.

While it was once difficult to buy medicinal herbs, it is now very easy to find the most popular ones at well-stocked pharmacies and even on the shelves of big-box stores. Health food stores offer an extensive selection of whole herbs, along with tinctures, teas, ointments, and other products that make it easy to skip pharmaceuticals.

It may come as a surprise to learn that a number of conventional pharmaceuticals have their roots firmly planted in herbal medicine. Aspirin comes from willow bark, and morphine is carefully compounded from opium poppies. Quinine, a vital drug for the treatment of malaria, comes from the bark of the cinchona tree, and digoxin, a potent drug used in cardiac cases, comes from the beautiful but poisonous foxglove. Many other pharmaceuticals are plant based or are synthesized using compounds that are identical to those found in nature.

Still, mainstream medicine prefers synthetic drugs for their standardization, purity, and ease of use. Understandably, prescription pharmaceuticals have earned a coveted status. It is not the intent of this book to downplay their importance. However, it's equally important to remember that in the United States, herbs are considered to be dietary supplements, and when sold commercially, they're regulated as such. Therefore, when you make the decision to treat an ailment the natural way, you don't need to obtain a prescription—as you would with a synthetic drug—to use an herbal poultice, apply a simple cream or oil, or take a tincture or tea.

While herbs are powerful, most do not have the lingering side effects that often accompany drugs. They do not inhibit the body's natural healing process; instead, they boost our ability to recover, particularly when paired with rest. Many herbs help boost the immune system, too, making it easier for the body to use its natural defenses against viruses and infections.

Cataloguing the world's medicinal plants would take an immense effort, and, even then, it would be nearly impossible to cover all the properties offered by each and every plant. While there are many wonderful and extensive guides detailing hundreds of herbs, it can be difficult to decide what to use—especially when there are so many options available.

This book is different. Within these pages, you'll find a guide to using some of the world's most common and effective medicinal herbs. All of them are easy to find online or at your local health food store. It's also quite likely that you can find some of them growing within a short distance of your front door. A few may even be hiding inside your spice cabinet! Whether you are new to the world of herbal medicine or have already begun experiencing the healing power of plants, you'll find this book useful. The main section of the book covers 75 common ailments, along with treatments for each. The final chapter features profiles of 40 herbs, including important precautions and notes for identifying and even growing them if you like.

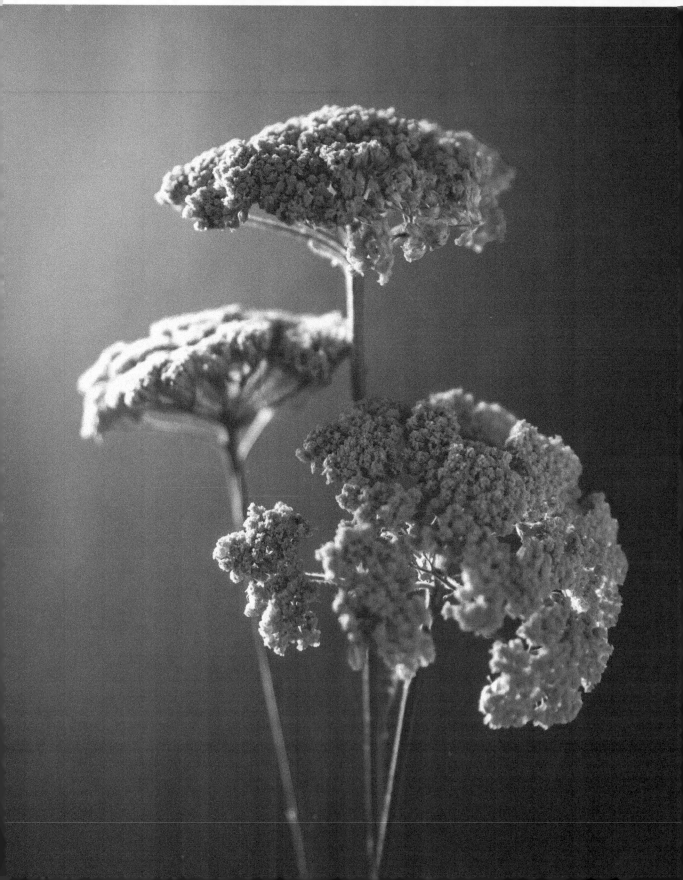

# CHAPTER 1

# Taking the Old and Making It New

*When you come down with a cold, it's convenient to reach for an over-the-counter treatment, but these can have adverse side effects. What's worse, many of us may be unknowingly over-medicating ourselves and our children, thinking that if a small dose of a drug is good, then more is even better. Herbal medicine provides a way to avoid the dangers of over-the-counter medicines, instead treating and healing common illnesses without all the synthetic ingredients. Whether you are experiencing insomnia, have a little one with itchy chicken pox, or find yourself dealing with an unexpected illness, it's likely that plant-based remedies can help.*

# Herbal Medicine in History

Before medications were manufactured by pharmaceutical companies, humans treated their ailments using what the earth provided. Whether this was an intuitive process or one discovered by trial and error, herbal medicine is not new. What *is* new is its resurgence, especially in the wake of well-publicized problems with mass-market drugs. But first, let's go back to the beginning. Almost every culture used local flora to develop their own plant-based remedies, and, thanks to each continent's varied ecosystem, people in different countries relied on unique remedies made with their native plants. Even today, modern medicines and treatments are inaccessible in many areas around the world, so herbal healers continue to play a crucial public health role.

## Africa

The oldest written medical texts date back thousands of years. Named the *Edwin Smith Papyrus* and *Papyrus Ebers* after the men who found them, these ancient Egyptian works include extensive descriptions of anatomy, notes on injuries, and information on herbal pharmacology, along with designs for medical and surgical instruments.

Traditional African medicine places an emphasis on herbal remedies, relying on a natural pharmacy that contains approximately 4,000 native plants. Even pharmaceutical companies recognize the importance of Africa's herbal medicines, learning from local practitioners and using traditional remedies to identify bioactive agents that can be used to prepare modern synthetic medicines.

## Asia

Early literature describing the use of Chinese herbs was found in Changsha, China, at the Mawangdui Han tombs that were sealed in 168 BCE. Called *Wushi'er Bingfang,* or *Recipes for 52 Ailments,* this list of prescriptions provides over 250 cures for ailments ranging from hemorrhoids to warts.

Traditional Asian medicine includes massage, exercise, acupuncture, and herbal treatments, along with dietary therapy. These practices were standardized in China during the 1950s but date back to about 1100 BCE, when dozens of herbal remedies were described. By the end of the sixteenth century, traditional Asian physicians had approximately 1,900 remedies at their disposal, and by the end of the twentieth century, the Chinese materia medica contained 12,800 different drugs.

In India, a major sourcebook called the *Atharva Veda* laid down the principles of

Ayurveda, a healing practice that began around 1200 BCE. This system is still in use today.

Ancient Middle Eastern physicians were learned herbalists who taught Greek and Persian scholars. Later, Arabs shared their knowledge with European crusaders, who in turn brought it back to their own countries.

## Australia

Although Australia was first visited by European ships in the 1600s, indigenous and imperialist cultures collided in 1788 when Britain's First Fleet brought about 1,500 people to Sydney.

At the time, aboriginal people relied heavily on herbal medicine. However, because their culture uses oral history—storytelling, singing, and dancing rituals—to pass down information, there are no written records of Australia's earliest herbal medicines. As the last remaining practicing elders pass away, fewer rituals take place, and more information concerning the continent's medicinal flora is lost.

Today, indigenous aboriginal medicine is referred to as *bush medicine*. The practice centers around traditional treatments utilizing Australian leaves and seeds. Native grapes and banksia flowers are also considered to be valuable local treatments, while eucalyptus and turmeric are prized worldwide.

This book allows you to take your health into your own hands, but sometimes modern medical care is necessary. Use these treatments wisely and judiciously—if you have a prolonged medical issue, please see a doctor.

## Europe

Early Greek and Roman physicians were renowned for their herbal knowledge. Much of what they knew had been passed down from Egyptian physicians. Often referred to as "the father of medicine," Hippocrates studied under Egyptian priest-doctors.

When the Roman Empire fell, scientific progress came to a halt, and much understanding of herbal medicine was lost. As trade with other civilizations increased, though, knowledge of medicinal herbs grew again. During the Renaissance, European nobles attempted to curate all human knowledge in vast libraries; in their gardens, they made impressive efforts to assemble the most useful botanicals of the time. During the sixteenth and seventeenth centuries, universities taught herbalism and botany, planting "physic" (or herb) gardens containing favorite medicinal plants.

In 1652, Nicholas Culpeper published *The English Physician*, a comprehensive herbal catalog of England's known herbal remedies. The book was meant for common people, with an emphasis on using herbs to heal common maladies instead of using expensive concoctions prepared by doctors.

As the scientific age dawned, the popularity of herbal remedies waned. Herbal remedies were nearly forgotten with the advent of modern drugs but are once again gaining popularity throughout Europe.

## North America

Native American and First Nations people have been using nature's medicines for tens of thousands of years, focusing on healing the body as well as purifying the spirit and balancing the mind. Oral traditions passed down through the ages indicate that the first healers learned how to use medicinal herbs by observing sick animals. Because information was passed via word of mouth, there are no written records of how native North Americans used herbs before their first contact with Europeans. However, this changed as indigenous people shared their natural remedies with the new settlers, many of whom brought with them knowledge of European herbal medicine. Indeed, many colonists brought their favorite healing plants with them to the New World.

A number of these plants have naturalized throughout North America and can be found growing alongside the continent's native flora.

As time passed, herbal remedies were largely replaced with drugs similar to those used in Europe. But in some places, including Appalachia, Alaska, Hawaii, and remote tribal lands in the western United States and Canada, herbal medicine remains a mainstay.

## South America

Central and South American natives used medicinal plants extensively. Shamanic traditions continue today, using the same plant medicines that have been revered for thousands of years. This continent is home to a vast number of plants with many medicinal uses, and traditional healers, or *yerbaristes,* can be found selling their remedies at market stalls. Many forest workers spend weeks at a time deep in the jungle, and rely heavily on plants for food, medicine, and materials to build shelters.

The herbal knowledge that still exists in remote jungle locations is vast. Ancient Mayan and Aztec healers had long used a variety of treatments made with healing plants. They also maintained hospitals where sick people were isolated from the rest of their community while receiving the care and attention they needed.

Today, cities, plantations, and ranches occupy South American land once bursting with native flora. Still, South America offers a wealth of medicinal plants in its deep jungles. New species are discovered frequently, highlighting both the need for conservation and the potential for promising treatments for conditions like malaria and cancer.

## UNUSUAL HISTORICAL TREATMENTS

History is filled with tales of bizarre natural medicinal practices. Here are 10 of the most unusual.

- During the medieval period, burns were soothed by applying slime from a live snail.

- Ancient Egyptians used a combination of macerated mice and other ingredients to ease the pain of a toothache.

- Snake oil was an actual treatment, not just a euphemism as it is today. For centuries, oil extracted from the fat of Chinese water snakes was used as a remedy for joint pain. Some traditional Chinese medical practitioners still recommend it.

- Thomas Edison, Pope Leo XIII, and Queen Victoria are a few famous figures who enjoyed a brew called Vin Mariani, which was red wine infused with coca leaves (the raw material used to manufacture cocaine).

- During the Middle Ages, many doctors believed that "like cures like." They recommended that people store their own flatulence in jars, to be sniffed from whenever the stench of the Black Death entered their neighborhoods.

- A seventeenth-century book of medical advice tells parents to soothe teething babies by cutting the foot off a live mole and then hanging it around the child's neck.

- The first saliva to enter the mouth on waking, also known as "fasting spittle," was once used to treat eye inflammation, ringworm, and warts.

- An old-fashioned gout treatment involved whipping oneself with stinging nettles until the skin was blistered and inflamed. Wealthy sufferers could pay a doctor to whip them or have a servant administer the treatment.

- One eighteenth-century French doctor recommended that his patients gargle with urine to cure dental maladies.

- During the late Victorian and early Edwardian eras, doctors recommended that their asthma patients swallow either a live, buttered frog or a handful of live spiders.

# Modern (Herbal) Medicine

Today, herbal medicine makes use of traditional treatments as well as standardized herbal extracts. Plants are being assessed for their pharmacological qualities, and as knowledge grows, individuals are better able to care for themselves. Many communities are home to naturopaths and well-educated herbal practitioners. High-quality supplements are easy to find in stores and online, making it easy to incorporate herbal medicine into your everyday life.

**Herbal medicine lets you avoid pharmaceuticals unless you truly need them.** Drugs often come with unpleasant or dangerous side effects, while herbal medicine provides gentler relief. If you do need an antibiotic for a particularly nasty infection, it will work better if you haven't previously been taking antibiotics for every minor runny nose and earache.

**Plant-based remedies cost less.** Who doesn't want to save money? Once you purchase or grow the plant material you need, you'll find that your cost per treatment drops dramatically.

**Botanicals help you feel healthier, naturally.** Many herbal remedies offer multiple benefits so you feel healthier overall while obtaining relief from your itchy eczema, irritating sniffles, or upset stomach.

**Many herbal remedies are family friendly.** Many herbs are safe for the whole family to use. With a few basic tools and ingredients, plus know-how and planning, you can treat minor illnesses naturally—and keep doctor visits to a minimum.

# Care and Cultivation

This book focuses more on remedies and application, so you'll primarily find resources on what ingredients you need and where to buy them. But for those of you with green thumbs, here's some information on growing, maintaining, and harvesting healing herbs.

## Plant a Healthy Landscape

Many medicinal plants do more than treat your family's minor ailments; they can also attract pollinators while adding beautiful colors to your home's landscape. Focus on perennial plants, and you'll have fewer gardening chores to tend to each year. Some excellent perennials to consider include echinacea, bee balm, catnip, and lavender. If you happen to have migraines, be sure to include some feverfew in your perennial herb garden.

# OF NATURAL ORIGIN

Many common medicines are rooted in herbal practices or are derived from plant life. The more you learn about herbal medicine, the more you'll discover. For now, here are seven of more than a hundred active ingredients that come from plants.

- Atropine, a medication used for a variety of purposes including bradycardia and heart block, comes from deadly nightshade, *Atropa belladonna*.

- Berberine, a treatment for dysentery, comes from the common barberry, *Berberis vulgaris*.

- Codeine and morphine, two powerful painkillers, come from a strain of poppy called *Papaver somniferum*.

- Digitalin, digitoxin, and digoxin are three cardiac drugs that come from the purple foxglove, *Digitalis purpurea*.

- Reserpine, an antihypertensive and antipsychotic drug, comes from the Indian snakeroot, *Rauvolfia serpentina*.

- Rhomitoxin, a tranquilizer and antihypertensive medication, comes from the rhododendron, *Rhododendron molle*.

- Theobromine, which is used as a stimulant, vasodilator, and diuretic, comes from the cocoa plant, *Theobroma cacao*.

## Prepare Those (Garden) Beds

Make sure your medicinal plants stay their healthiest by preparing a place for them to grow before you bring them home. Follow planting instructions precisely, and keep a close eye on them during the first week after transplanting, as they may need extra water or some protection from hot sun until they settle in.

## Save Your Pennies

American ginseng and goldenseal are two examples of very useful herbs that are traditionally gathered from their natural habitats in a practice called *wildcrafting*, where uncultivated herbs, plants, and even fungi are gathered from the wild,

then replanted at home for new harvests. If there's a certain herb that you enjoy using and would prefer to stop paying for, learn about its needs and consider growing it in your garden. You can find seeds and rootstock online.

## Plan Ahead

Learn as much as you can about the plants you plan to harvest from nature, and look for them before harvest time so that you'll be able to watch them and make your harvest at the best possible time. Be sure that wildcrafting is allowed in the place where you plan to harvest your herbs, and obtain any necessary permits before removing even a single plant.

## Get Educated

Many medicinal herbs are considered to be weeds; the dandelion is a prime example. You can safely wildcraft at home by keeping your lawn organic and encouraging plants like mullein, low-growing plantain, chickweed, and dandelion to mingle with your grass. Allow them to grow, harvest what you want, and then mow as usual. These hardy herbs will return each year with no effort on your part. Protect yourself by gathering herbs only in areas where no herbicide or pesticide has been applied.

# The Science behind the Remedies

We've learned that many herbs and botanicals form the basis for some common medications. As we explore the remedies, we'll get into this in more detail, but here's an essential explanation of what's at work when you use herbal remedies.

## Gastrointestinal Health and Good Liver Function

Minor digestive complaints such as indigestion and nausea often respond well to herbal remedies. A cup of peppermint or chamomile tea is sometimes all that's needed to help you feel more comfortable. Overburdened livers benefit, too, as many herbs provide protection and can even help restore normal function following injury or illness. Milk thistle is a well-known example of an herb that can help keep your liver healthy.

## Immune Function, Infection, and Inflammation

Many botanical medicines benefit your immune system, while others help your body stave off infection and fight inflammation. Echinacea is an example of an immune-stimulant herb that helps prevent infection, while ginseng is a botanical that can boost the immune system and help you maintain good health. St. John's wort, ginger, and ginkgo biloba are some of the best botanicals for reducing inflammation.

## Musculoskeletal Discomfort

Minor sprains, sore muscles, and painful joints can be targeted with internal and external herbal medicines. Internally, botanicals with high levels of antioxidants support connective tissue health; externally, herbs like calendula, witch hazel, and capsicum provide soothing comfort.

## Psychological, Neurological, and Behavioral Health

Watch an advertisement for prescription drugs that aim to improve mental health, and you'll notice that most of them come with warnings concerning potential side effects. Herbal remedies like ginkgo biloba and valerian can make a positive difference in restoring balance without causing their own problems.

## Reproductive Health

Premenstrual syndrome (PMS), menopause symptoms, and pregnancy side effects are often easier to manage when you know which herbs to use. Ginger can help you deal with morning sickness, and both PMS and menopause symptoms respond well to black cohosh. Ginseng, ginkgo biloba, and saw palmetto are a few of the herbs that support the male reproductive system.

## Respiratory Health

Sore throats, coughs, and colds are often treated with over-the-counter medications that cause uncomfortable side effects. However, these irritations often respond well to herbal medicines, as do stuffy sinuses and minor respiratory infections. Echinacea plays a starring role in cold and flu treatments, while thyme and hyssop can help relieve bronchial spasms so you can rest.

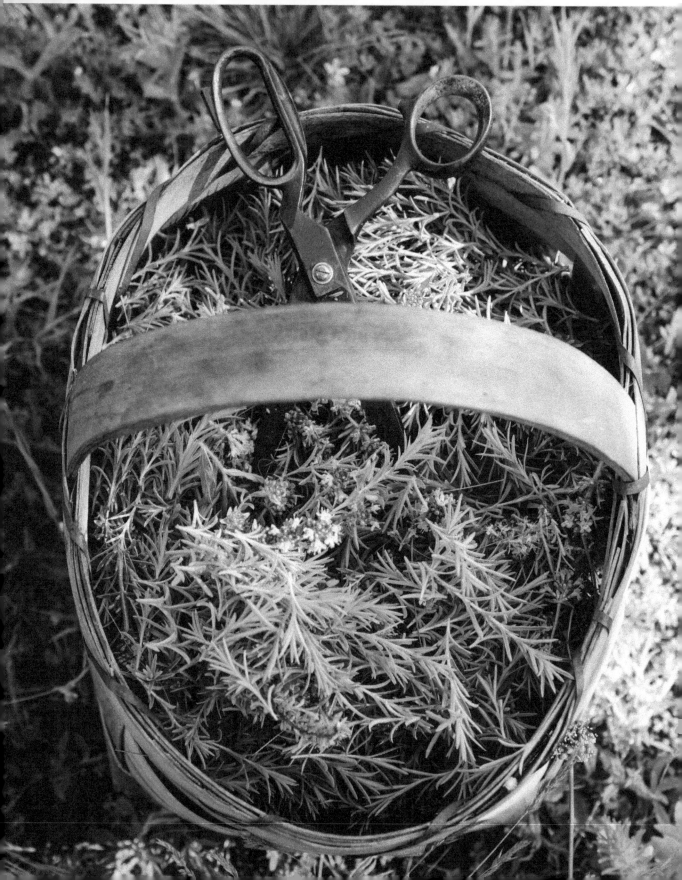

# CHAPTER 2

# The Herbal Kitchen

*If you're comfortable in the kitchen, then you're well on your way to making herbal medicines, and you may already have some of the essentials on hand. If you're not much of a chef, don't worry—it's easy to learn how to make your own medicines at home. From stocking up on the right tools and ingredients to working safely, this chapter sets you up for success.*

# A Well-Stocked Pantry

Correct preparation of each remedy is key to ensuring effectiveness. Here are some items that are not plant life, but are still necessary tools for your herbal medicine journey.

## Kitchen and Cookware

- Pots and pans; preferably not aluminum or Teflon
- Double boiler
- Drying racks; preferably not aluminum or Teflon
- Mixer
- Blender or food processer
- Tea kettle
- Ceramic teapot with a lid
- Kitchen scale
- Glass or ceramic bowls in varying sizes
- Strainers in at least three different sizes
- Funnels
- Utensils such as measuring cups, spoons, spatulas, and whisks

## Storage and Use

- Cosmetic jars and tins with tight-fitting lids
- Large, medium, and small glass canning jars with tight-fitting lids
- Large, medium, and small glass bottles with tight-fitting lids
- Medium and small dark-colored glass bottles with dropper tops
- Labels for your ingredients and remedies (simple masking tape will do in a pinch)
- Cotton balls or cosmetic pads

## Shopping Tips

- Don't worry about buying all your supplies brand-new. You can sterilize and recycle jars and bottles, especially ones with interesting shapes, to showcase your remedies.
- Buying in bulk will save you money; consider purchasing more supplies than you actually need.
- Shop around to get the best prices on essentials such as fingertip sprayers, lotion bottles with pump tops, lip balm tubes, and more. You can often find a wide variety of containers at the same health food stores and online shops that carry medicinal herbs.
- Keep an eye out for interesting packaging items if you plan to give herbal remedies as gifts.
- Make detailed notes about your suppliers. This way, you'll know exactly where to buy what you need when you find yourself running low in the future.

# Methods of Application and Necessary Tools

Herbal medicines can be taken internally and applied externally, and there are a variety of ways to deliver treatments. This section offers a general overview.

## Boluses

Boluses are suppositories meant for rectal or vaginal use. Because they melt at body temperature, it's best to make them in a cool environment. Work quickly, and refrigerate the boluses as soon as they are finished. Boluses will keep for three to six weeks in the refrigerator.

- Nonreactive saucepan
- Shallow baking pan
- Plastic wrap
- Wax paper
- Whisk and spatula
- Glass bowl
- Glass or plastic storage container with a tight-fitting lid
- Coconut oil or pure cocoa butter
- Powdered herbs

## Creams, Lotions, Balms, and Salves

Creams, lotions, balms, and salves can stay fresh for up to a year. Although some recipes can be labor-intensive, the results are well worth the work. Since these recipes are not intended for consumption and are usually used up quickly, you can store them in just about any container that has been scrubbed clean and run through the dishwasher. Check each recipe to see which tools you'll need; the following are sure to be useful.

- Double boiler
- Mixer
- Mixing bowls
- Whisks, spoons, and spatulas
- Dried herbs or infused oils
- Essential oils (optional)
- Lotion bases, waxes, and oils

## Decoctions

Decoctions—extractions involving mashing and then boiling an herb in water to extract oils, organic compounds, or essential chemicals—are suitable for making poultices, or concentrating and adding to syrups.

- Nonreactive saucepan or stockpot with a lid
- Sterilized glass bottle or jar for storage
- Cheesecloth
- Dried herbs
- Water

## Infused Oils

While infused oils can be used on their own, they are also essential for making balms and salves. Be sure that your herbs are completely dry before using them to make infused oil; any moisture will cause mold that will spoil the entire batch. The shelf life of infused oils depends on the shelf life of the oil type. Almond oil, for example, has a 1-year shelf life when kept in a cool, dark place.

- Sterilized jar with a tight-fitting top
- Sterilized glass bottle or jar for storage
- Cheesecloth
- Slow cooker or oven (or even a sunny windowsill)
- Dried herbs
- Essential oils (optional)
- Oil

## Liniments

Liniments are alcohol- or oil-based herbal extracts that are meant to be applied to the skin. Like alcohol-based tinctures, liniments offer the advantage of a 7- to 10-year shelf life.

- Sterilized jar with a tight-fitting top
- Sterilized glass bottle or jar for storage
- Cheesecloth
- Dried herbs
- Essential oils (optional)
- Vodka, vinegar, or apple cider vinegar

## Teas and Infusions

Teas and infusions are quick and easy to prepare, since they contain only herbs and water. While these remedies are typically ingested, they can also be sprayed on or applied with a poultice. Like decoctions, teas and infusions may be concentrated and compounded into syrups. When sealed and stored in a cool, dark place, dry teas have a 1- to 4-year shelf life.

- Tea kettle or saucepan
- Ceramic teapot with lid
- Mugs or cups
- Fresh or dried herbs
- Empty teabags for premeasured teas
- Infuser for loose leaf teas
- Sterilized glass bottle or jar for storage

## Tinctures

Tinctures, or infused extracts, offer a cost-effective method for concentrating and preserving herbs. Alcohol-based tinctures have an average shelf life of 7 to 10 years, while those made with glycerin will last up to 3 years when refrigerated. Tinctures made with apple cider vinegar have a 3- to 6-month shelf life when stored in the refrigerator, so plan to use them up shortly after making them.

- Glass jar with a tight-fitting lid (pint size or larger)
- Sterilized bottle or jar for storage (preferably dark-colored glass bottles with dropper tops)
- Cheesecloth
- Dried herbs
- Unflavored 80-proof vodka
- Food-grade vegetable glycerin or apple cider vinegar for alcohol-free tinctures

# OTHER NECESSARY INGREDIENTS

With a fairly modest selection of ingredients, you can easily produce a wide variety of creams, balms, salves, and other products.

- Natural **beeswax** is essential for solidifying salves, hardening balms, and making long-lasting body products that provide protection while nourishing skin. It is sold in solid form as well as in convenient pastilles that measure easily and melt quickly.

- **Carnuba wax** comes from a Brazilian palm tree. It is a plant-based alternative to beeswax and is used in the same way.

- Solid **cocoa butter** adds a thick, rich, creamy consistency to salves, creams, and lotions. Pressed from roasted cacao seeds, it has a light, almost chocolaty aroma. Cocoa butter softens at body temperature, so it's very easy to melt and blend with other ingredients. You can find it in jars and convenient pastilles or wafers.

- **Coconut oil** is a very accessible addition to your herbal kitchen. Its antimicrobial properties make it an excellent base for healing salves. It is a solid at room temperature, whereas fractionated coconut oil remains a liquid at room temperature and has a longer shelf life.

- **Essential oils** aren't a traditional part of herbal medicine, but because many of them come from medicinal plants and are readily accessible, they make a perfect addition to your recipes.

- **Honey** is an excellent preservative for syrups, and it makes unpalatable herbs far easier to swallow. Vegans, babies, and people who are allergic to honey can use simple sugar syrup instead.

- **Jojoba oil** is a liquid plant wax with a very light, nongreasy feel. It often costs more than vegetable and nut oils do, but it has a longer shelf life and greater stability. Its average shelf life is 3 years at room temperature or 4 years in the refrigerator.

- **Olive oil** makes an excellent base for infused oils, and it's very easy to find high-quality organic olive oil at most supermarkets. Choose a light olive oil rather than a virgin one if you prefer a less noticeable aroma.

- Thanks to its ability to deliver intense moisture, **shea butter** is a favorite ingredient in lotions and creams. It makes a wonderful addition to healing salves, too. If you dislike the aroma of shea butter, you'll be glad to know that it is available in a naturally deodorized formula with a far more subtle fragrance. You can substitute mango or cocoa butter in recipes that call for shea.

## Poultices

A poultice can be as simple as crushed fresh herbs applied to a rash or bug bite, or a quick compress made with a clean, folded cloth.

- Clean tea towel, bandage, cheesecloth, or reusable muslin bag
- Fresh or dried herbs
- Water or apple cider vinegar

## Powders and Caplets

Powdered herbs form the basis for caplets, and they are also useful for making body powders, adding to bath products, and imparting flavor to foods. When sealed and stored in a dark, cool environment, powders and caplets have a shelf life of 1 to 4 years. It's best to make small batches if you don't plan to use your herbs frequently; the longer they spend in storage, the less potent they become.

- Coffee grinder, herb grinder, blender, food processer, or mortar and pestle
- Dark-colored glass jar with a tight-fitting lid
- Empty vegetable gel capsules and encapsulating device
- Fine-mesh strainer

# Practicing Safely

While many people believe that herbal medicines are completely safe because they come from plants, some herbs are deadly. Others should be used infrequently, and some can interact with one another or with prescription medications. Protect yourself and your family by confirming that herbs are safe to use under your unique set of circumstances.

## Herbs to Avoid at All Times

Remember to stay safe by avoiding any herbs you cannot positively identify. Some herbs should be avoided outright. This is by no means an exhaustive list, as there are countless poisonous plants.

- Belladonna
- Daffodil
- Foxglove
- Hemlock
- Henbane
- Jimsonweed
- Mandrake
- Tansy
- Wolfsbane

## Herbs to Avoid During Pregnancy and Lactation

Like other substances, the constituents in herbs are passed on to your baby when you ingest them. Many herbs stimulate the uterus and can cause contractions, while others affect hormone levels. This is by no means an exhaustive list, and you should always check to ensure that herbs are safe to take when you are pregnant or breastfeeding.

- Angelica
- Basil
- Black cohosh
- Catnip
- Comfrey
- Feverfew
- Goldenseal
- Mistletoe
- Mugwort
- Pennyroyal
- Rosemary
- Yarrow

## Guidelines for Treating Babies and Toddlers

Infants and toddlers can safely take many herbal remedies, but be sure to double-check that treatments are safe before you administer them. Here are a few general guidelines:

- Children under age two respond best to mild remedies like chamomile, peppermint, dandelion, slippery elm, and catnip.
- You can use stevia to sweeten herbal teas for children who need to avoid sugar, especially those too young to ingest honey. (Never give honey to a baby under the age of one because of the risk of he or she ingesting botulism spores.)
- Children under age two do not have fully developed livers, and thus have a hard time breaking down alcohol and pungent plants. Before giving an alcohol-based tincture to a young child (or to anyone else who should avoid

alcohol), add a drop of the tincture to a cup of boiling water. The alcohol will have evaporated completely by the time the water is cool enough to drink.

## Herbs to Avoid with Heart Medication

If you take prescription drugs for heart disease, there are certain herbs you should avoid. This list includes several that can cause serious interactions, but there are many others you should research.

- Alfalfa
- Aloe vera
- Bilberry
- Black cohosh
- Echinacea
- Garlic
- Ginkgo biloba
- Hawthorn
- Licorice root
- Saw palmetto
- St. John's wort
- Yohimbe

## Herbs to Avoid with Medical Conditions

Certain herbs are restricted from use at the same time as prescription medicines, and others are not suitable for use in people with medical conditions. Here are just a few examples.

- Do not take St. John's wort if you take warfarin, protease inhibitors, certain asthma drugs, oral contraceptives, or antidepressants.
- Evening primrose increases seizure risk in people with epilepsy.

- Garlic, ginger, ginkgo biloba, fever-few, and evening primrose can increase bleeding risk in people with bleeding disorders and in those who take blood thinners.
- If you take immunosuppressant drugs such as methotrexate, azathioprine, cyclosporine, or any corticosteroids such as prednisone, avoid alfalfa, astragalus, echinacea, licorice root, and ginseng. Because these herbs stimulate the immune system, they may counteract your prescribed medication.

## Carefully Purchasing Herbs

Although herbs are not regulated like pharmaceuticals, they can be just as potent. Be sure that the herbs, plants, and seeds you buy come from a reliable source. Packages should be clearly labeled, and safety information should be readily available. Avoid sources that paint all herbs with the same brush by making statements that all plants are natural, safe, and effective. If something seems too good to be true, it probably is.

## Appropriately Packaging Herbs

You might wonder why glass jars and bottles are recommended for the long-term storage of your herbal remedies, especially when so many of the raw ingredients you buy come in plastic packages. Plastic bottles, jars, and bags are used for shipping, since they prevent breakage and weigh less than glass. Certain plastic packages can leach chemicals into the contents inside, so storing your herbs in glass helps ensure purity.

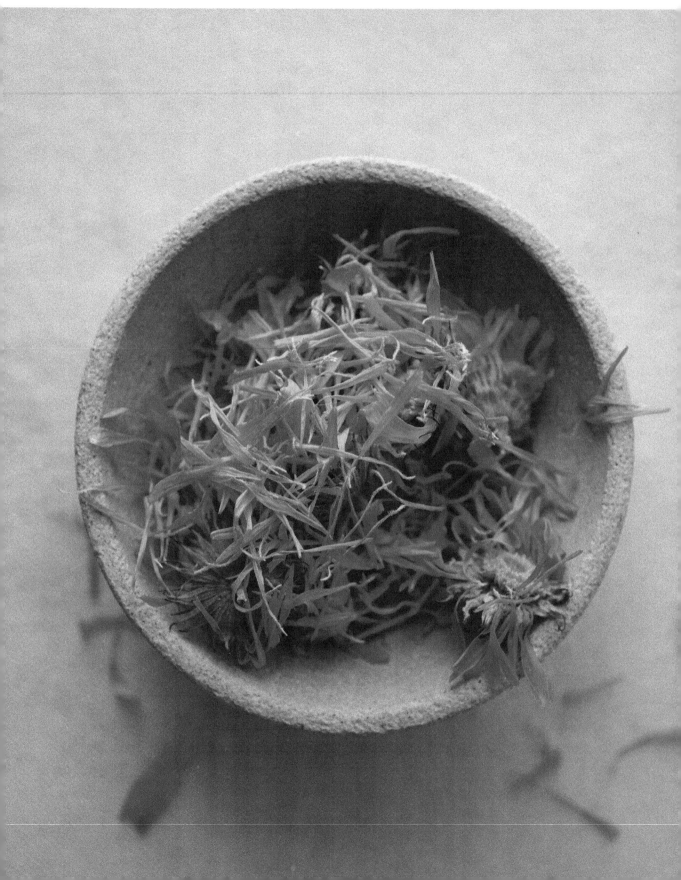

# CHAPTER 3

# Remedies and Recipes

*Everyday ailments can be easy to treat with basic recipes, simple kitchen tools, and a well-stocked pharmacy of herbs. Whether you have been stung by a bee while tending your tomatoes or hit by a flying baseball at your child's Little League game, you'll find a long list of useful remedies here.*

# Abscess

*Painful and hot to the touch, an abscess is an inflamed or infected area filled with pus. The larger an abscess grows, the more painful it becomes. You should seek medical attention if herbal remedies don't help, since the infection inside a large abscess can spread to surrounding tissue and into the bloodstream.*

## Fresh Yarrow Poultice

### Makes 1 poultice

Yarrow contains anti-inflammatory and antibacterial compounds. It works by disinfecting the abscess, easing swelling, and promoting faster healing.

1 tablespoon finely chopped fresh yarrow leaves

1. Apply the chopped leaves to the abscess, then cover with a soft cloth. Leave the poultice in place for 10 to 15 minutes.
2. Repeat two or three times per day until the abscess is healed.

**Precautions** Do not use during pregnancy. Yarrow can cause skin reactions in people who are allergic to plants in the Asteraceae family.

# Echinacea and Goldenseal Tincture

Makes about 2 cups

Echinacea and goldenseal offer strong anti-bacterial benefits, plus they boost your natural immune response. Make this tincture ahead of time so you have it on hand when you need it. Stored in a cool, dark place, it will last for up to 7 years. Use it any time you have an infection.

5 ounces dried echinacea root, finely chopped

3 ounces dried goldenseal root, finely chopped

2 cups unflavored 80-proof vodka

1. In a sterilized pint jar, combine the echinacea and goldenseal. Add the vodka, filling the jar to the very top and covering the herbs completely.
2. Cap the jar tightly and shake it up. Store it in a cool, dark cabinet and shake it several times per week for 6 to 8 weeks. If any of the alcohol evaporates, add more vodka so that the jar is again full to the top.
3. Dampen a piece of cheesecloth and drape it over the mouth of a funnel. Pour the tincture through the funnel into another sterilized pint jar. Squeeze the liquid from the roots, wringing the cheesecloth until no more liquid comes out. Discard the roots and transfer the finished tincture to dark-colored glass bottles.
4. To treat an abscess, take 10 drops orally two or three times a day for 7 to 10 days.

**Precautions** Do not use during pregnancy. Use caution if you have diabetes, as goldenseal can sometimes lower blood sugar.

# Acne

*Red and inflamed, infected seba-*
*ceous glands create painful pimples.*
*While this condition usually affects*
*teens, adults can get it, too. Whether*
*the acne affects only your face or has*
*spread to your chest, back, or other*
*body parts, herbal remedies help you*
*look and feel better.*

## Calendula Toner

Makes about ½ cup

With soothing calendula that addresses
inflammation, this simple toner also contains witch hazel, which targets bacteria
while softening your skin. When kept in a
cool, dark place, this toner stays fresh for
at least a year.

2 tablespoons calendula oil

⅓ cup witch hazel

1. In a dark-colored glass bottle, combine
   the ingredients and shake gently.
2. With a cotton cosmetic pad, apply 5 or
   6 drops to your freshly washed face or
   other areas of concern. Use a little more
   or less as needed.
3. Repeat twice per day while acne persists.
   Store the bottle in the refrigerator if you
   think you'd like a cooling sensation.

# Agrimony-Chamomile Gel

**Makes about ⅔ cup**

Agrimony and chamomile, combined with aloe vera gel, soothe redness and ease inflammation. Store the gel in the refrigerator. When kept an airtight container, it will remain fresh for up to 2 weeks.

2 teaspoons dried agrimony

2 teaspoons dried chamomile

½ cup water

¼ cup aloe vera gel

1. In a saucepan, combine the agrimony and chamomile with the water. Bring the mixture to a boil over high heat, then reduce the heat to low. Simmer the mixture until it reduces by half, then remove it from the heat and allow it to cool completely.

2. Dampen a piece of cheesecloth and drape it over the mouth of a funnel. Pour the mixture through the funnel into a glass bowl. Squeeze the liquid from the herbs, wringing the cheesecloth until no more liquid comes out.

3. Add the aloe vera gel to the liquid and use a whisk to blend. Transfer the finished gel to a sterilized glass jar. Cap the jar tightly and store it in the refrigerator.

4. With a cotton cosmetic pad, apply a thin layer to all affected areas twice a day.

**Precautions** Omit the chamomile if you take prescription blood thinners or are allergic to plants in the ragweed family.

# Allergies

*Allergies are abnormal immune responses to a common substance such as cat dander, pollen, or dust. Allergens are found in food, drinks, and the environment, so it's often difficult to avoid them completely. Whereas conventional treatments suppress your body's immune response to allergens that affect you, herbal remedies are far gentler.*

## Feverfew-Peppermint Tincture

Makes about 2 cups

Feverfew and peppermint open up the airways during an allergy attack. If you must stay away from feverfew, make this tincture with peppermint alone. The tincture will keep for up to 7 years in a cool, dark place.

2 ounces dried feverfew

6 ounces dried peppermint

2 cups unflavored 80-proof vodka

1. In a sterilized pint jar, combine the feverfew and peppermint. Add the vodka, filling the jar to the very top.
2. Cap the jar tightly and shake it up. Store it in a cool, dark cabinet and shake it several times per week for 6 to 8 weeks.
3. Dampen a piece of cheesecloth and drape it over the mouth of a funnel. Pour the tincture through the funnel into another sterilized pint jar. Wring the liquid from the herbs. Discard the spent herbs and transfer the finished tincture to dark-colored glass bottles.
4. Take 5 drops orally whenever allergy symptoms flare up. If the taste is too strong for you, you can mix it into a glass of water or juice and drink it.

**Precautions** Do not use feverfew if you are allergic to ragweed. Do not use feverfew during pregnancy.

# Garlic-Ginkgo Syrup

Makes about 2 cups

Ginkgo biloba is a natural antihistamine that contains more than a dozen anti-inflammatory constituents, while garlic bolsters your immune system. Use local honey if possible, as it can help build resistance to allergens that are found in your area. This syrup will stay fresh for up to 6 months when refrigerated.

2 ounces fresh or freeze-dried garlic, chopped

2 ounces ginkgo biloba, crushed or chopped

2 cups water

1 cup local honey

1. In a saucepan, combine the garlic and ginkgo biloba with the water. Bring the liquid to a simmer over low heat, cover partially with a lid, and reduce the liquid by half.
2. Transfer the contents of the saucepan to a glass measuring cup, then pour the mixture through a dampened piece of cheesecloth back into the saucepan, wringing the cheesecloth until no more liquid comes out.
3. Add the honey and warm the mixture over low heat, stirring constantly and stopping when the temperature reaches 105°F to 110°F.
4. Pour the syrup into a sterilized jar or bottle and store it in the refrigerator.
5. Take 1 tablespoon orally three times per day until your allergy symptoms subside.

**Precautions** Do not use if you are taking a monoamine oxidase inhibitor (MAOI) for depression. Ginkgo biloba enhances the effect of blood thinners, so talk to your doctor before use. Children under age 12 should take 1 teaspoon three times per day.

# Asthma

*This chronic ailment involves inflamed airways throughout the lungs, along with constricted bronchial tubes. Asthma attacks can be very frightening, so some people also experience panic attacks when breathing becomes difficult.*

## Ginkgo-Thyme Tea

Makes 1 cup

Ginkgo biloba and thyme help open your airways and relax the muscles in your chest so that you can breathe easier. If you dislike the flavor of this tea, you can add a teaspoon of honey or dried peppermint to the blend to improve its taste.

1 cup boiling water

1 teaspoon dried ginkgo biloba

1 teaspoon dried thyme

1. Pour the boiling water into a large mug. Add the dried herbs, cover the mug, and allow the tea to steep for 10 minutes.
2. Relax and drink the tea slowly while inhaling the steam. Repeat up to four times per day.

**Precautions** Do not use if you are taking a monoamine oxidase inhibitor (MAOI) for depression. Ginkgo biloba enhances the effect of blood thinners, so talk to your doctor before use.

# Peppermint-Rosemary Vapor Treatment

Makes 1 treatment

Peppermint helps open your airways and ease breathing, while rosemary leaves contain essential histamine-blocking oil. If you don't have fresh herbs available for this treatment, you can replace them with 2 drops of peppermint essential oil and 4 drops of rosemary essential oil.

4 cups steaming-hot water (not boiling)

½ cup crushed fresh peppermint leaves

½ cup finely chopped fresh rosemary leaves

1. In a large, shallow bowl, combine all the ingredients. Place the bowl on a table and seat yourself comfortably in front of it.
2. Use a large towel to cover your head and the bowl. Breathe the vapors that rise from the herbs. Emerge for fresh air as needed, and close your eyes if the vapors feel too strong. Continue the treatment until the water has cooled.
3. Repeat as needed whenever asthma symptoms arise. This treatment is gentle enough to use as often as you like.

**Precautions** Do not use rosemary if you have epilepsy. Although some calming oils like jasmine, ylang-ylang, chamomile, and lavender have been shown to prevent seizures, more-pungent oils like rosemary, fennel, sage, eucalyptus, hyssop, camphor, and spike lavender have been known to trigger epileptic incidents.

# Athlete's Foot

*This itchy, sometimes painful infection is caused by a fungus that thrives in moist, warm, dark places. Be sure to treat it before it gets under your toenails, where it will cause discoloration and disfigurement that are very difficult to eradicate.*

## Fresh Garlic Poultice

Makes 1 treatment

Garlic is a very strong antifungal agent that kills athlete's foot. Raw honey helps bind the garlic to your feet while providing additional antifungal activity. While it's possible to make a double or triple batch of this remedy and use it over the course of 2 to 3 days, you may achieve faster healing by making a fresh batch for each individual treatment.

1 garlic clove, pressed

1 teaspoon raw honey

1. In a small bowl, combine the garlic and honey. With a cotton cosmetic pad, apply the blend to the affected area.
2. Put on a pair of clean socks and relax with your feet up, leaving the poultice in place for 15 minutes to an hour. Wash and dry your feet afterward. Repeat the treatment once or twice per day, and follow up with an application of Goldenseal Ointment (following page). Continue for 3 days after symptoms disappear.

**Precautions** Garlic may cause a skin rash in sensitive individuals.

# Goldenseal Ointment

Makes about 1 cup

Goldenseal is a potent antimicrobial agent that helps put a stop to athlete's foot. You can use this ointment on its own, or speed healing by using it in concert with a Fresh Garlic Poultice (previous page). It will stay fresh for up to a year when stored in a cool, dark place.

1 cup light olive oil

2 ounces dried goldenseal root, chopped

1 ounce beeswax

1. In a slow cooker, combine the olive oil and goldenseal. Select the lowest heat setting, cover the slow cooker, and allow the roots to steep in the oil for 3 to 5 hours. Turn off the heat and allow the infused oil to cool.

2. Bring an inch or so of water to a simmer in the base of a double boiler. Reduce the heat to low.

3. Drape a piece of cheesecloth over the upper half of the double boiler. Pour in the infused oil, then wring and twist the cheesecloth until no more oil comes out. Discard the cheesecloth and spent herbs.

4. Add the beeswax to the infused oil and place the double boiler on the base. Gently warm over low heat. When the beeswax melts completely, remove the pan from the heat. Quickly pour the mixture into clean, dry jars or tins and allow it to cool completely before capping.

5. With a cotton cosmetic pad, apply ¼ teaspoon to each affected area. Use a little more or less as needed, and repeat up to three times per day, with the final application being before bed. Wear a pair of clean socks over the ointment to prevent slipping.

**Precautions** Do not use if you are pregnant or breastfeeding. Do not use if you have high blood pressure.

# Backache

*While most back pain is preceded by overwork or an injury, it is sometimes caused by inactivity, muscle spasms, or inflammation. Rest as much as you can to speed healing, and be sure to see your doctor if the pain is severe or if it is accompanied by numbness, tingling, or incontinence.*

## Passionflower-Blue Vervain Tea

Makes 1 cup

Both passionflower and blue vervain relax the nervous system and soothe sore muscles. This is a deeply relaxing blend, so be sure to take it when you have some time to rest.

1 cup boiling water

1 teaspoon dried passionflower

1 teaspoon dried blue vervain

1.  Pour the boiling water into a large mug. Add the dried herbs, cover the mug, and allow the tea to steep for 10 minutes.
2.  Relax and drink the tea slowly. Repeat up to two times per day.

**Precautions** Do not use passionflower or blue vervain during pregnancy. Avoid passionflower if you have prostate problems or baldness.

# Ginger-Peppermint Salve

## Makes about 1 cup

Ginger and peppermint contain potent constituents that penetrate the skin, creating a warming sensation that promotes muscle relaxation. This salve will remain fresh for up to a year when stored in a cool, dark place.

1 cup light olive oil

1 ounce dried gingerroot, chopped

1 ounce dried peppermint, crushed

1 ounce beeswax

1. In a slow cooker, combine the olive oil, ginger, and peppermint. Select the lowest heat setting, cover the slow cooker, and allow the herbs to steep in the oil for 3 to 5 hours. Turn off the heat and allow the infused oil to cool.

2. Bring an inch or so of water to a simmer in the base of a double boiler. Reduce the heat to low.

3. Drape a piece of cheesecloth over the upper half of the double boiler. Pour in the infused oil, then wring and twist the cheesecloth until no more oil comes out. Discard the cheesecloth and spent herbs.

4. Add the beeswax to the infused oil and place the double boiler on the base. Gently warm over low heat. When the beeswax melts completely, remove the pan from the heat. Quickly pour the mixture into clean, dry jars or tins and allow it to cool completely before capping.

5. Using your fingers or a cotton cosmetic pad, apply 1 teaspoon to the affected area, massaging well. Use a little more or less as needed. Repeat the treatment up to four times per day.

**Precautions** Do not use ginger if you take prescription blood thinners, have gallbladder disease, or have a bleeding disorder.

# Bee Sting

*Pain, redness, and swelling often accompany a bee sting, and the discomfort can last long after the actual event. Herbs help ease the pain. However, if you are allergic to bee venom, remember that herbal treatments are not intended to replace emergency EpiPens.*

## Fresh Plantain Poultice

Makes 1 treatment

The humble plantain plant—not to be confused with its banana-like namesake—is a green weedy plant containing a glucoside called aucubin, a potent antitoxin. Other constituents offer antiseptic and anti-inflammatory benefits, making this simple treatment incredibly effective. If you can't find fresh plantain leaves, you can soak a teaspoon of dried, crushed plantain in a tablespoon of water to rehydrate it for use as a poultice.

1 tablespoon finely chopped fresh
  plantain leaves

Apply the chopped leaves to the affected area and cover with a soft cloth. Leave the poultice in place for 10 to 15 minutes. Repeat as often as needed until the pain stops permanently.

# Comfrey-Aloe Gel

Makes about ¼ cup

Comfrey's anti-inflammatory and analgesic properties give it the ability to ease the pain and swelling that accompany bee stings. Aloe provides cool comfort and speeds healing. If you like this balm, you'll find it useful for a variety of little cuts and scrapes. When kept in the refrigerator, it stays fresh for about 2 weeks.

2 teaspoons dried comfrey

¼ cup water

2 tablespoons aloe vera gel

1. In a saucepan, combine the comfrey and water. Bring the mixture to a boil over high heat, then reduce the heat to low. Simmer the mixture until it reduces by half, then remove it from the heat and allow it to cool completely.

2. Dampen a piece of cheesecloth and drape it over the mouth of a funnel. Pour the mixture through the funnel into a glass bowl. Squeeze the liquid from the comfrey, wringing the cheesecloth until no more liquid comes out.

3. Add the aloe vera gel to the liquid and use a whisk to blend. Transfer the finished gel to a sterilized glass jar. Cap the jar tightly and store it in the refrigerator.

4. With a cotton cosmetic pad, apply a thin layer to the affected area as often as needed until the pain and swelling subside.

# Bloating

*Overeating, abdominal gas, and the onset of women's premenstrual cycles are a few of the things that can bring on an uncomfortable bout of bloating. Herbs help your body return to a more balanced state by supporting the elimination of toxins, excess gas, and built-up fluid.*

## Peppermint-Fennel Tea

Makes 1 cup

If you suspect that your bloating is caused by buildup in your digestive tract, you'll find that peppermint and fennel provide comfort and quick relief. These pleasant-tasting plants contain strong antispasmodic agents that relax smooth muscle tissue in the digestive tract. Add a teaspoon of honey if the flavor of this tea is too strong for you.

1 cup boiling water

1 teaspoon dried peppermint

¼ teaspoon fennel seeds, crushed

1. Pour the boiling water into a large mug. Add the peppermint and fennel, cover the mug, and allow the tea to steep for 10 minutes.
2. Relax and drink the tea. This is a mild remedy and can be repeated as often as needed.

# Dandelion Root Tincture

**Makes about 2 cups**

Dandelion root has a bitter taste, but it offers strong diuretic benefits that will help your body release toxins and make you feel far more comfortable. This tincture will remain fresh for up to 7 years if it is kept in a cool, dark place.

8 ounces dandelion root, finely chopped

2 cups unflavored 80-proof vodka

1. Put the dandelion root in a sterilized pint jar. Add the vodka, filling the jar to the very top and covering the roots completely.
2. Cap the jar tightly and shake it up. Store it in a cool, dark cabinet and shake it several times per week for 6 to 8 weeks. If any of the alcohol evaporates, add more vodka so that the jar is again full to the top.
3. Dampen a piece of cheesecloth and drape it over the mouth of a funnel. Pour the tincture through the funnel into another sterilized pint jar. Squeeze the liquid from the roots, wringing the cheesecloth until no more liquid comes out. Discard the roots and transfer the finished tincture to dark-colored glass bottles.
4. Take 1 teaspoon orally once or twice per day whenever bloating is a problem. If the taste is too strong for you, you can mix it into a glass of water or juice and drink it.

# Bronchitis

*Often the result of irritation, infection, or allergies, bronchitis occurs when the bronchial linings become inflamed. The condition is also usually characterized by a deep, rasping cough. Herbal treatments, combined with increased fluid intake and plenty of rest, have proven useful in reducing and eliminating the symptoms of bronchitis.*

## Rosemary-Licorice Root Vapor Treatment

Makes 1 treatment

Rosemary and licorice root help open the airways, stimulate circulation, and ease the discomfort and inflammation that often accompany bronchitis.

5 cups water

¼ cup chopped dried licorice root

½ cup finely chopped fresh rosemary leaves

1. In a saucepan, combine the water and the dried licorice root. Bring the mixture to a boil and then reduce the heat to low. Simmer for 10 minutes.
2. Pour the water and licorice root into a shallow bowl and add the rosemary leaves.
3. Use a large towel to cover your head and the bowl. Breathe in the vapors that rise from the herbs. Emerge for fresh air as needed, and close your eyes if the vapors feel too strong. Continue the treatment until the water has cooled.
4. Repeat as needed. This treatment is gentle enough to use as often as you like.

**Precautions** Do not use this treatment if you have epilepsy, high blood pressure, diabetes, kidney problems, or heart disease.

# Goldenseal-Hyssop Syrup

Makes about 2 cups

Goldenseal contains two strong antiviral and antibacterial agents called hydrastine and berberine. Hyssop eases bronchial spasms and helps clear lung congestion while imparting a soothing, calming effect that will help you relax. This syrup is also good for treating the common cold. It will keep for up to 6 months when refrigerated.

½ ounce dried goldenseal root, chopped

1 ounce dried hyssop

2 cups water

1 cup honey

1. In a saucepan, combine the goldenseal and hyssop with the water. Bring the liquid to a simmer over low heat, cover partially with a lid, and reduce the liquid by half.
2. Transfer the contents of the saucepan to a glass measuring cup, then pour the mixture though a dampened piece of cheesecloth back into the saucepan, wringing the cheesecloth until no more liquid comes out.
3. Add the honey and warm the mixture over low heat, stirring constantly and stopping when the temperature reaches 105°F to 110°F.
4. Pour the syrup into a sterilized jar or bottle and store it in the refrigerator.
5. Take 1 tablespoon orally three to five times per day until your symptoms subside.

**Precautions** Do not use if you are pregnant or breastfeeding. Do not use if you have epilepsy or high blood pressure. Goldenseal can aggravate diarrhea and heartburn. Children under age 12 should take 1 teaspoon two to three times per day.

# Bruise

*Deep, painful bruises can be indicative of other injuries or health complications. Minor bruises can be caused by something as simple as bumping into a piece of furniture. If you suddenly start bruising more easily than usual, see your doctor, as consistent bruising can be an indication of an underlying health issue.*

## Fresh Hyssop Poultice

**Makes 1 treatment**

Hyssop offers pain relief and stimulates circulation, helping your bruise heal faster. If you haven't yet added hyssop to your garden, you can use a drop or two of hyssop essential oil to treat a bruise. You can also rehydrate a teaspoon of dried hyssop with a tablespoon of warm water and use it to make a poultice.

1 tablespoon finely chopped fresh
　hyssop leaves

Apply the chopped leaves to the affected area and cover with a soft cloth. Leave the poultice in place for 10 to 15 minutes. Repeat two or three times per day until your bruise fades.

**Precautions** Hyssop can produce sudden and involuntary muscle contractions, so it should not be used if you have epilepsy or are pregnant.

# Arnica Salve

Makes about 1 cup

Arnica is a strong anti-inflammatory agent, and its ability to relieve pain makes this simple salve an excellent choice for bumps and bruises.

1 cup light olive oil

2 ounces dried arnica flowers

1 ounce beeswax

1. In a slow cooker, combine the olive oil and arnica. Select the lowest heat setting, cover the slow cooker, and allow the herbs to steep in the oil for 3 to 5 hours. Turn off the heat and allow the infused oil to cool.
2. Bring an inch or so of water to a simmer in the base of a double boiler. Reduce the heat to low.
3. Drape a piece of cheesecloth over the upper half of the double boiler. Pour in the infused oil, then wring and twist the cheesecloth until no more oil comes out. Discard the cheesecloth and spent herbs.
4. Add the beeswax to the infused oil and place the double boiler on the base. Gently warm over low heat. When the beeswax melts completely, remove the pan from the heat. Quickly pour into clean, dry jars or tins and allow it to cool completely before capping.
5. With your fingers or a cotton cosmetic pad, apply a pea-size amount to the bruised area. Use a little more or less as needed, and repeat twice a day until your bruise fades.

**Precautions** Do not use on broken skin. Irritation can occur with long-term use; discontinue if signs of skin irritation appear.

# Burn

*Herbal remedies are suitable for minor burns such as those sustained while cooking. Seek immediate medical treatment for any burn that appears deep, involves charred skin, or covers a large part of the body.*

## Chickweed-Mullein Compress

### Makes 1 treatment

Mullein's antibacterial and anti-inflammatory properties prevent burns from becoming infected, and its cooling, astringent property helps ease the pain. Chickweed provides additional cooling power and helps speed the healing process.

2 teaspoons finely chopped chickweed

1 teaspoon finely chopped fresh mullein leaf

Apply the freshly chopped plant matter to the burn and surrounding area and cover with a soft cloth. Leave the poultice in place for 10 to 15 minutes. Repeat every 2 to 3 hours or more frequently, until the pain subsides.

# Fresh Aloe Vera Gel

Makes 1 treatment

Aloe vera gel contains antibacterial compounds that help prevent burns from becoming infected, and it also offers anti-inflammatory benefits. Aloe stimulates collagen synthesis, so skin regenerates faster after a minor burn. While it's strongest when taken fresh from the plant, bottled aloe gel will do in a pinch.

Aloe vera plant

1. Cut a 1-inch section from the tip of an aloe vera leaf. Leave the rest of the leaf on the plant, where it will continue to grow.
2. With a sharp knife, slit the leaf open. Use your fingers or a cotton cosmetic pad to scoop the gel from the center of the leaf and apply the entire amount to the burn and the surrounding area. Repeat once or twice per day while your burn is healing.

# Canker Sore

*A painful red blister that mysteriously appears inside the mouth, an occasional canker sore is irritating but not worth worrying about. See your doctor for testing if canker sores recur frequently, as they can be an indication of an underlying metabolic disorder.*

## Calendula-Comfrey Poultice

Makes 1 treatment

Soothing calendula offers antifungal, anti-inflammatory, and antibacterial properties, and it helps minor wounds heal faster. Comfrey helps speed healing, too, and it offers some relief from the pain and itching that accompany a canker sore. If you like this treatment, you can save time by multiplying it and making several dry poultices at once.

⅛ teaspoon dried calendula

⅛ teaspoon dried comfrey

2 tablespoons hot water

1. Use a mortar and pestle or grinder to reduce the herbs to a rough powder, then transfer the powder to a 2-inch square of muslin.
2. Fold the muslin into a small packet, enclosing the herbs. Place it in the hot water for 2 minutes.
3. Place the finished poultice inside your mouth with the thinnest layer of fabric against the canker sore. Leave it in place for 10 to 15 minutes. Repeat two or three times per day until the canker sore is gone.

# Goldenseal Tincture

Makes about ⅔ cup

The berberine and hydrastine in goldenseal root give this herb excellent value as a broad-spectrum antiviral and antibacterial agent. Besides using this goldenseal tincture on canker sores, you can use it to treat minor cuts, scrapes, and burns. You can also take it internally when you feel a cold or the flu coming on.

4 ounces dried goldenseal root, finely chopped

1 cup unflavored 80-proof vodka

1.  Put the goldenseal in a sterilized half-pint jar. Add the vodka, filling the jar to the very top and covering the roots completely.
2.  Cap the jar tightly and shake it up. Store it in a cool, dark cabinet and shake it several times per week for 6 to 8 weeks. If any of the alcohol evaporates, add more vodka so that the jar is again full to the top.
3.  Dampen a piece of cheesecloth and drape it over the mouth of a funnel. Pour the tincture through the funnel into another sterilized half-pint jar. Squeeze the liquid from the roots, wringing the cheesecloth until no more liquid comes out. Discard the roots and transfer the finished tincture to dark-colored glass bottles.
4.  With a cotton swab, dab 2 or 3 drops on the canker sore. Breathe through your mouth to avoid salivating while the tincture dries. Repeat two or three times per day until the canker sore disappears.

**Precautions** Do not use if you are pregnant or breastfeeding. Do not use if you have high blood pressure.

# Chapped Lips

*Sometimes painfully cracked, and others times rough and peeling, chapped lips aren't merely a cosmetic problem. Chapping often happens because the lips are not able to produce their own moisture. Exposure to sun, wind, heating, and air conditioning can make things worse, as can licking your lips in an attempt to moisturize them and alleviate your discomfort.*

## Aloe-Calendula Balm

Makes 2 tablespoons

Aloe vera and calendula help compromised skin heal, and aloe brings deeply penetrating moisture to thirsty lips. This quick recipe makes use of premade calendula oil; however, you can replace it with infused calendula oil you've crafted on your own. When refrigerated and tightly capped, this balm will stay fresh for up to a year.

1½ tablespoons aloe vera gel

1½ teaspoons calendula oil

1.  In a small bowl, combine the aloe vera gel and calendula oil. With a whisk, blend them thoroughly.
2.  Transfer the balm to a container with a tight-fitting lid. While it's best to keep your main supply refrigerated so that it stays fresh, you may want to carry a teaspoon or so along in a small squeeze bottle so that you can apply it throughout the day.
3.  With your fingertip or a cotton swab, apply a thin layer to your lips. Just a drop or two at a time should be enough; reapply as needed throughout the day and again at bedtime.

# Comfrey-Hyssop Lip Balm

Makes about ⅔ cup
(enough to fill 10 lip balm tubes)

Both comfrey and hyssop offer anti-inflammatory and analgesic properties, helping compromised skin heal faster while providing some relief from the discomfort that accompanies chapped lips. You can easily halve or double this recipe. The finished product will stay fresh for about a year when kept in a cool, dark place.

2 tablespoons jojoba oil

1 tablespoon cocoa butter

1 tablespoon light olive oil

1 teaspoon dried comfrey

1 teaspoon dried hyssop

4 teaspoons grated beeswax or
    beeswax pastilles

3 drops vitamin E oil (optional)

1. Bring an inch or so of water to a simmer in the base of a double boiler. Reduce the heat to low.

2. In a glass measuring cup, combine the jojoba oil, cocoa butter, olive oil, and herbs. Place the measuring cup in the upper part of the double boiler and allow it to gently warm over low heat for 2 to 3 hours. Check the water level in the base of the double boiler occasionally to ensure that it has not evaporated.

3. Drape a piece of cheesecloth over a small bowl and pour the infused oil through it. Wring and twist the cheesecloth until no more oil comes out. Discard the cheesecloth and spent herbs.

4. Return the infused oil to the measuring cup and add the beeswax. Return the measuring cup to the top of the double boiler and gently warm over low heat until the beeswax has melted.

5. Remove the measuring cup from the double boiler and add the vitamin E oil (if using). Immediately pour the mixture into clean, dry lip balm tubes or tins and allow to cool completely before capping.

6. Apply a thin layer of balm to your lips as often as needed throughout the day and just before going to sleep at night.

**Precautions** Omit the hyssop and double the comfrey if you are pregnant or have epilepsy.

# Chest Congestion

*When you're having trouble breathing, herbs can help ease your lungs and make you more comfortable while you address the cause of your congestion.*

## Hyssop-Sage Infusion

Makes 1 quart

Hyssop is a strong antiviral, plus an effective expectorant. Sage contributes its antiseptic property, helping you heal faster. This blend has a strong herbal taste that some people like; others find that they need to add a little bit of honey to make it go down easier.

4 cups boiling water

4 teaspoons dried hyssop

4 teaspoons dried sage

1. In a teapot, combine the boiling water and dried herbs. Cover the pot and allow the infusion to steep for 10 minutes.
2. Relax and drink a cup of the infusion slowly while inhaling the steam. You can reheat or refrigerate the rest and sip it over the course of the day.

**Precautions** Do not take hyssop if you are pregnant or have epilepsy.

# Angelica-Goldenseal Syrup

Makes about 2 cups

Angelica relieves congestion by stimulating and warming the lungs while alleviating some of the associated discomfort. Goldenseal offers strong antiseptic and antiviral properties, helping you get over your illness faster. Honey masks the bitter flavors while coating your throat, which might be a bit sore from any associated coughing. This syrup stays fresh for up to 6 months when refrigerated.

1 ounce angelica, finely chopped

1 ounce dried goldenseal root, finely chopped

2 cups water

1 cup honey

1. In a saucepan, combine the herbs and water. Bring the liquid to a simmer over low heat, cover partially with a lid, and reduce the liquid by half.
2. Transfer the contents of the saucepan to a glass measuring cup, then pour the mixture through a dampened piece of cheesecloth back into the saucepan, wringing the cheesecloth until no more liquid comes out.
3. Add the honey and warm the mixture over low heat, stirring constantly and stopping when the temperature reaches 105°F to 110°F.
4. Pour the syrup into a sterilized jar or bottle and store it in the refrigerator.
5. Take 1 tablespoon orally three or four times per day until your symptoms subside. Children under age 12 should take 1 teaspoon two or three times per day.

**Precautions** Do not use if you are pregnant or breastfeeding. Do not take angelica with anticoagulant drugs. Do not take goldenseal if you have high blood pressure.

# Chicken Pox

*A highly contagious infection, chicken pox brings an itchy, blistered rash with it. Nothing cures chicken pox, but herbal remedies can help ease the discomfort.*

## Comfrey-Licorice Bath

Makes 1 quart

Comfrey and licorice root soothe the itching of chicken pox while offering antiviral benefits. The apple cider vinegar has a pungent smell, but it adds even more soothing power. This quick recipe makes use of pre-made comfrey and licorice root tinctures, but you can easily replace them with home-made ones.

4 cups organic unfiltered apple cider vinegar

½ teaspoon comfrey tincture

½ teaspoon licorice root tincture

1. In a clean, dry jar, combine the vinegar and tinctures. Cap tightly and store in a cool, dark place until ready to use.
2. Draw a lukewarm bath and add 1 cup of the blend to the water. Spend at least 20 minutes soaking. Repeat once or twice per day, and follow up with the Calendula-Goldenseal Gel (following page) if desired.

**Precautions** Do not use licorice root if you have high blood pressure, diabetes, kidney problems, or heart disease.

# Calendula-Goldenseal Gel

Makes about 2 cups

Aloe, calendula, and goldenseal combine to soothe itching and irritation while helping chicken pox blisters heal. This gel is a good one for other rashes and skin irritations, such as minor cuts and scrapes. It will stay fresh for up to 2 weeks when refrigerated.

1 ounce dried calendula

1 ounce dried goldenseal root, chopped

2 cups water

1½ cups aloe vera gel

1. In a saucepan, combine the calendula and goldenseal with the water. Bring the mixture to a boil over high heat, then reduce the heat to low.
2. Simmer the mixture until only about ½ cup remains, then remove it from the heat and allow it to cool completely.
3. Dampen a piece of cheesecloth and drape it over the mouth of a funnel. Pour the mixture through the funnel into a glass bowl. Squeeze the liquid from the herbs, wringing the cheesecloth until no more liquid comes out.
4. Add the aloe vera gel to the liquid and use a whisk to blend. Transfer the finished gel to a sterilized glass jar. Cap the jar tightly and store it in the refrigerator.
5. With a cotton cosmetic pad, apply a thin layer to all affected areas two or three times per day.

**Precautions** Do not use if you are pregnant or breastfeeding. Do not use if you have high blood pressure.

# Cold

*With symptoms that include coughing, sneezing, and a sore throat, the common cold can be a drag. Shorten your cold's duration by beginning treatment as soon as symptoms appear.*

## Thyme Tea

Makes 1 cup

Thyme acts as an antitussive, or cough suppressant, quickly calming coughing. It pulls double duty by acting as an expectorant that clears congestion from the lungs. It also soothes the pain of a sore throat and relieves the body aches that often accompany a cold. Add a teaspoon of honey to this tea if you prefer a sweet flavor.

1 cup boiling water

2 teaspoons dried thyme

1. Pour the boiling water into a large mug. Add the thyme, cover the mug, and allow the tea to steep for 10 minutes.
2. Relax and drink the tea slowly while inhaling the steam. Repeat up to six times per day.

# Herbal Cold Syrup with Comfrey, Mullein, and Raspberry Leaf

Makes about 2 cups

Comfrey helps coughs and sore throats, while mullein, thyme, and raspberry leaf address fever, body aches, and lung irritation. Don't worry too much if you're missing one or two of the herbs used in this recipe; all of them are beneficial and will ease your cold symptoms. This syrup stays fresh for up to 6 months when refrigerated.

½ ounce dried comfrey

½ ounce dried mullein

½ ounce dried raspberry leaf

½ ounce dried thyme

2 cups water

1 cup honey

1. In a saucepan, combine the herbs and water. Bring the liquid to a simmer over low heat, cover partially with a lid, and reduce the liquid by half.
2. Transfer the contents of the saucepan to a glass measuring cup, then pour the mixture through a dampened piece of cheesecloth back into the saucepan, wringing the cheesecloth until no more liquid comes out.
3. Add the honey and warm the mixture over low heat, stirring constantly and stopping when the temperature reaches 105°F to 110°F.
4. Pour the syrup into a sterilized jar or bottle and store it in the refrigerator.
5. Take 1 tablespoon orally three or four times per day until your symptoms subside. Children under age 12 should take 1 teaspoon two or three times per day.

**Precautions** Never use raspberry leaves that are not completely dried, as fresh ones can cause nausea.

# Cold Sore

*Caused by the herpes simplex virus, cold sores appear in the mouth and on the lips. It's best to apply herbal remedies at the first sign of tingling and itching, well before the raised clusters of blisters appear. If you already have an untreated cold sore, herbal remedies may not be strong enough to stop the virus from running its course, though they may provide soothing relief.*

## Garlic Poultice

Makes 1 treatment

Raw garlic has a pungent odor, but it is a strong antiviral agent that can help shorten the duration of a cold sore. If you don't like the idea of holding the garlic in place, you can try using a piece of first aid tape to hold it in place so that you can multitask.

1 garlic clove, cut in half

1. Wash and dry the affected area.
2. Apply the cut side of the garlic to the cold sore and hold it in place for 10 minutes. Repeat three or four times per day until the cold sore is gone.

**Precautions** Garlic can cause a skin rash in sensitive individuals; discontinue treatment if this occurs.

# Echinacea-Sage Toner

**Makes about ½ cup**

Echinacea and sage offer potent antiviral properties, plus antibacterial properties that help prevent the sores from becoming infected. The witch hazel and aloe help by easing the itching. This toner will stay fresh for at least a year when refrigerated.

½ ounce dried echinacea root, chopped

½ ounce dried sage, crumbled

2 tablespoons jojoba or light olive oil

2 tablespoons aloe vera gel

¼ cup witch hazel

1. In a slow cooker, combine the herbs and oil. Select the lowest heat setting, cover the slow cooker, and allow the herbs to steep in the oil for 3 to 5 hours. Turn off the heat and allow the infused oil to cool.
2. Drape a piece of cheesecloth over a bowl. Pour the infused oil through the cheesecloth, then wring and twist the cheesecloth until no more oil comes out. Discard the cheesecloth and spent herbs.
3. Transfer the infused oil to a dark-colored glass bottle, then add the aloe vera gel and witch hazel. Combine the ingredients by shaking gently.
4. With a cotton swab, apply 1 or 2 drops to the affected area. Use a little more or less as needed.
5. Repeat two or three times per day while the cold sore persists. Store the bottle in the refrigerator.

**Precautions** Omit the echinacea if you are allergic to ragweed or have an autoimmune disease.

# Colic

*A frustrating condition, colic affects infants between 2 weeks and 4 months of age. Bouts of crying that last for hours, sleeplessness, and inconsolability are among the most common symptoms. Herbal remedies don't prevent colic, since there are many causes; however, they can ease the pain.*

## Chamomile Infusion

Makes 1 cup

Chamomile contains a strong anti-spasmodic constituent, spiroether, which relaxes tense, aching muscles and helps relieve the pain of colic. Its ability to calm stress and anxiety can help your baby get the sleep he or she needs, too. If you're breastfeeding, you may find that drinking chamomile tea helps ease your baby's symptoms.

1 teaspoon dried chamomile

1 cup boiling water

1. In a teapot, combine the chamomile and the boiling water. Cover the pot and allow the tea to steep for 10 minutes. Allow the infusion to cool to lukewarm.
2. Transfer 2 tablespoons to a sterilized bottle and let your baby sip on it. Repeat once or twice per day whenever colic symptoms arise.

**Precautions** Do not use chamomile if you are taking prescription blood thinners.

# Herbal Gripe Water with Fennel, Ginger, and Peppermint

**Makes 1 cup**

Commercial gripe water often contains high-fructose corn syrup. This DIY version contains a little sugar, along with fennel, ginger, and peppermint, and helps relieve discomfort by relaxing the intestinal muscles and releasing trapped gas. This remedy will keep for a week when refrigerated.

1 teaspoon crushed fennel seeds

1 teaspoon chopped fresh gingerroot

1 teaspoon crushed dried peppermint leaves

1 cup boiling water

1 teaspoon cane sugar

1. In a teapot or mug, combine the herbs and boiling water. Cover the pot or mug and allow the blend to steep for 10 minutes.
2. Transfer the gripe water to a sterilized jar with a tight-fitting lid. Add the sugar and stir until it dissolves. Allow the gripe water to cool to lukewarm.
3. Transfer 1 teaspoon to a medicine dropper and gently administer it orally to your baby. Repeat once or twice per day whenever colic symptoms arise.

**Precautions** Omit the ginger if your baby has a bleeding disorder.

# Conjunctivitis

*Redness, itching, crusting or discharge, and tearing of the eyes are all symptoms of conjunctivitis. Also known as pinkeye, this common complaint can cause dry eyes, puffy eyelids, and sensitivity to light.*

## Quick Chamomile Poultice

### Makes 1 treatment

Chamomile soothes the pain and itch of conjunctivitis while also offering anti-inflammatory and antibacterial benefits. Plain chamomile tea bags, preferably organic, make this treatment a very simple one to use in a hurry.

¼ cup steaming-hot (not boiling) water
1 organic chamomile tea bag

1. Put the water in a small cup or bowl and submerge the tea bag in it. Allow it to sit for 2 minutes.
2. Remove the tea bag from the water and allow it to cool until it is hot but comfortable to touch. Close the affected eye and relax. Press the tea bag lightly against your eye and leave it in place for 10 to 20 minutes. Replace two or three times per day while recovering from conjunctivitis.

**Precautions** Do not use if you are allergic to plants in the ragweed family or take prescription blood thinners.

# Goldenseal Poultice

Makes 1 treatment

Thanks to its ability to soothe irritation while fighting inflammation and infection, goldenseal is an excellent treatment for conjunctivitis. If you like this treatment, you can save time by preparing several poultices in advance and then activating them with hot water when you are ready to use them.

½ cup steaming-hot water (not boiling)

1 tablespoon chopped dried goldenseal root

1. Pour the hot water into a small bowl. Put the chopped goldenseal root in a reusable linen bag and place the bag in the hot water. Allow the poultice to sit in the water for 5 to 10 minutes, or until the roots soften.

2. Close your eye and relax. Press the poultice lightly against your eye and leave it in place for 10 to 20 minutes. Repeat two or three times per day while recovering from conjunctivitis.

**Precautions**  Do not use if you are pregnant or breastfeeding. Do not use if you have high blood pressure.

# Constipation

*Abdominal pain and difficult bowel movements are among the top symptoms of constipation. Herbs provide effective relief while being far easier on your system than harsh chemical laxatives. Help things move faster by upping your fiber intake, drinking plenty of water, and increasing physical activity.*

## Aloe Vera Juice

**Makes about 3 cups**

Aloe vera juice improves digestion and sweeps the digestive tract clean. This makes it perfect for treating chronic constipation. Freshly made aloe juice should be consumed within 3 days.

1 fresh 3- to 4-inch aloe leaf from the inner portion of the plant

3 cups fresh juice, water, or coconut water

1. Hold the aloe leaf upside down over the sink so that the resin drips away from where you cut it. When the resin stops dripping, cut the leaf in half lengthwise and carefully scoop out the gel from the inside.
2. Put the gel in a blender and cover it with the liquid. Blend well, chill, and then enjoy. Drink 1 cup per day and store the leftovers in the refrigerator in a tightly covered bottle or jar.

**Precautions** Do not take aloe internally if you are pregnant or breastfeeding.

# Dandelion-Chickweed Syrup

Makes about 2 cups

Both dandelion and chickweed are gentle laxatives that alleviate constipation without harsh chemicals. You may be able to find both of these herbs in your own backyard; just be sure that neither has been contaminated with herbicide or chemical fertilizer. This syrup stays fresh for up to 6 months when refrigerated.

1 ounce dandelion root, chopped

1 ounce fresh or dried chickweed

2 cups water

1 cup honey

1. In a saucepan, combine the dandelion root, chickweed, and water. Bring the liquid to a simmer over low heat, cover partially with a lid, and reduce the liquid by half.
2. Transfer the contents of the saucepan to a glass measuring cup, then pour the mixture through a dampened piece of cheesecloth back into the saucepan, wringing the cheesecloth until no more liquid comes out.
3. Add the honey and warm the mixture over low heat, stirring constantly and stopping when the temperature reaches 105°F to 110°F.
4. Pour the syrup into a sterilized jar or bottle and store it in the refrigerator.
5. Take 1 tablespoon orally three or four times per day until your symptoms subside. Children under age 12 should take 1 teaspoon two or three times per day.

# Cough

*Coughing is one of the body's natural mechanisms for expelling irritants and excess phlegm buildup from the lungs and airways. What begins as an irritating itch in your throat can become worse if it persists—a dry, hacking, and unproductive cough. Herbal remedies soothe sensitive throat tissues while you address the underlying cause.*

## Fennel-Hyssop Tea

Makes 1 cup

Fennel loosens phlegm, making coughs more productive. If you have a dry, hacking cough and an irritated throat, you'll find that the fennel and hyssop in this tea provide quick relief from the discomfort.

1 cup boiling water

1 teaspoon fennel seeds

1 teaspoon dried hyssop

1. Pour the boiling water into a large mug. Add the herbs, cover the mug, and allow the tea to steep for 10 minutes.
2. Relax and drink the tea slowly while inhaling the steam. Repeat up to four times per day.

**Precautions** Do not take hyssop if you are pregnant or have epilepsy.

# Licorice-Thyme Cough Syrup

Makes about 2 cups

Licorice root is an excellent anti-inflammatory that quickly soothes irritated tissue inside the throat, while thyme acts as an expectorant that clears the lungs. Thyme is also an antitussive, a drug that calms coughing spasms. This cough syrup stays fresh for 6 months when refrigerated.

1 ounce licorice root, chopped

1 ounce thyme

2 cups water

1 cup honey

1. In a saucepan, combine the licorice root, thyme, and water. Bring the liquid to a simmer over low heat, cover partially with a lid, and reduce the liquid by half.
2. Transfer the contents of the saucepan to a glass measuring cup, then pour the mixture through a dampened piece of cheesecloth back into the saucepan, wringing the cheesecloth until no more liquid comes out.
3. Add the honey and warm the mixture over low heat, stirring constantly and stopping when the temperature reaches 105°F to 110°F.
4. Pour the syrup into a sterilized jar or bottle and store it in the refrigerator.
5. Take 1 tablespoon orally three or four times per day until your symptoms subside. Children under age 12 should take 1 teaspoon two or three times per day.

**Precautions** Do not take licorice if you have high blood pressure, diabetes, kidney problems, or heart disease.

# Cuts and Scrapes

*Minor injuries that don't require stitches can heal faster with a little help from herbs. Be sure to wash and dry the affected area before you apply any remedies.*

## Fresh Comfrey Poultice

Makes 1 treatment

Comfrey eases pain and is a strong anti-inflammatory that also offers anti-bacterial benefits. It contains a compound called allantoin that helps wounds heal faster. Honey is also an effective anti-bacterial agent, and in this recipe, it helps bind the comfrey to your skin. If you don't have fresh comfrey, you can use plantain, which also contains allantoin.

1 teaspoon crushed fresh comfrey

1 teaspoon honey

1. In a small bowl, use a fork to combine the honey and comfrey.
2. Wash and dry the injured area, then use a gauze pad to apply the poultice. Leave the gauze in place, cover it with a second piece of gauze, and secure it to the injured area with first aid tape.
3. Remove the poultice after an hour and gently rinse the injury with fresh, cool water to remove the stickiness and plant matter. Repeat two or three times per day as needed.

# Plantain Salve

Makes about 1 cup

Plantain is a wonderfully effective addition to your first aid arsenal. Offering quick relief from pain, it also boasts antibacterial compounds. Make this salve ahead of time so you'll have it when you need it; when kept in a cool, dark area, it stays fresh for up to a year.

4 ounces dried plantain

1 cup light olive oil

1 ounce beeswax

1. In a slow cooker, combine the plantain and olive oil. Select the lowest heat setting, cover the slow cooker, and allow the herbs to steep in the oil for 3 to 5 hours. Turn off the heat and allow the infused oil to cool.

2. Bring an inch or so of water to a simmer in the base of a double boiler. Reduce the heat to low.

3. Drape a piece of cheesecloth over the upper half of the double boiler. Pour in the infused oil, then wring and twist the cheesecloth until no more oil comes out. Discard the cheesecloth and spent herbs.

4. Add the beeswax to the infused oil and place the double boiler on the base. Gently warm over low heat. When the beeswax melts completely, remove the blend from the heat. Quickly pour the salve into clean, dry jars or tins and allow it to cool completely before capping.

5. With your fingers or a gauze pad, apply 1 teaspoon to the injured area. Use a little more or less as needed, ensuring that the entire injury is covered in a thin, protective layer. Repeat as often as needed.

# Dandruff

*Sometimes caused by a fungal infection or scalp psoriasis, dandruff causes an unpleasantly itchy and flaky scalp. However, it often responds well to gentle herbal treatments.*

## Echinacea Spray

Makes about 1 cup

Echinacea attacks candida, which is often to blame in severe cases of dandruff, and witch hazel helps put a stop to the itching. If your scalp is damaged from itching, the witch hazel will help it heal. This spray stays fresh for up to a year in the refrigerator.

1 cup witch hazel

2 tablespoons echinacea tincture

1. In a dark-colored glass bottle with a spray top, combine the ingredients. Shake gently to blend completely.
2. Apply 1 or 2 spritzes to each part of your scalp where dandruff is a concern. Massage the spray in with your fingertips, then brush or comb your hair. You can style your hair as usual and leave the spray in all day if you like, or you can leave it in for 1 to 2 hours and then shampoo it out. Use daily for best results.

**Precautions** Do not use echinacea if you have an autoimmune disorder or are allergic to ragweed.

# Rosemary Conditioner

## Makes 1 cup

This very simple antifungal remedy combines a natural, unscented conditioner designed for your specific hair type with rosemary essential oil, which is highly concentrated and wonderfully fragrant. If you don't have rosemary essential oil, you can use tincture in its place.

1 cup natural, unscented herbal conditioner like Stonybrook Botanicals

40 drops rosemary essential oil

1. In a large bowl, combine the conditioner with the essential oil, using a whisk or a fork to blend well. Use a funnel to transfer it to a BPA-free plastic bottle with a squeeze top.

2. After shampooing, apply a nickel-size dollop of conditioner to your scalp, using a little more or less as needed to cover it completely. Wait 2 to 5 minutes, then rinse the conditioner out with cool water. Style your hair as usual. Use daily for best results.

**Precautions** Do not use rosemary if you have epilepsy.

# Diaper Rash

*Diaper rash—accompanied by pain, redness, and swelling—can occur even when you are diligent about changing your baby's diaper. Herbal remedies are gentle enough for your baby's tender skin, and they contain none of the harmful talc or petroleum products found in many commercial preparations.*

## Chamomile-Echinacea Gel

Makes about ½ cup

Aloe, chamomile, and echinacea come together to heal and soothe your little one's rash. Echinacea targets yeast, a naturally occurring fungus that can make diaper rash worse. This gel stays fresh for up to 2 weeks when stored in the refrigerator.

1 tablespoon dried chamomile

1 tablespoon chopped dried echinacea root

½ cup water

¼ cup aloe vera gel

1.  In a saucepan, combine the chamomile and echinacea with the water. Bring the mixture to a boil over high heat, then reduce the heat to low. Simmer the mixture until it reduces by half, then remove it from the heat and allow it to cool completely.
2.  Dampen a piece of cheesecloth and drape it over the mouth of a funnel. Pour the mixture through the funnel into a glass bowl. Wring the cheesecloth until no more liquid comes out.
3.  Add the aloe vera gel to the liquid and use a whisk to blend. Transfer the finished gel to a sterilized glass jar. Cap the jar tightly and store it in the refrigerator.
4.  With a cotton cosmetic pad, apply a thin layer to all affected areas after each diaper change. Allow the gel to absorb completely and follow up with Comfrey-Thyme Salve (following page) before re-diapering. Continue to use this gel for at least 3 days after the diaper rash is gone.

**Precautions** Do not use echinacea if your baby has an autoimmune disorder.

# Comfrey-Thyme Salve

Makes about 1 cup

Comfrey helps speed healing, while thyme acts as a strong antibacterial agent. This rich salve also provides a barrier against moisture so your baby's skin has a chance to heal. Consider making a double batch; keep one jar in the diaper bag and another near your home changing area. This salve will last for a year in a cool, dark place.

1 cup light olive oil

1 ounce dried comfrey

1 ounce dried thyme

1 ounce beeswax

1. In a slow cooker, combine the olive oil, comfrey, and thyme. Select the lowest heat setting, cover the slow cooker, and allow the herbs to steep in the oil for 3 to 5 hours. Turn off the heat and allow the infused oil to cool.

2. Bring an inch or so of water to a simmer in the base of a double boiler. Reduce the heat to low.

3. Drape a cheesecloth over the upper half of the double boiler. Pour in the infused oil, then wring and twist the cheesecloth until no more oil comes out. Discard the cheesecloth and spent herbs.

4. Add the beeswax to the infused oil and place the double boiler on the base. Gently warm over low heat. When the beeswax melts completely, remove the pan from the heat. Quickly pour the salve into clean, dry jars or tins and allow it to cool completely before capping.

5. With your fingers or a gauze pad, apply a thin layer to your baby's diaper area after each diaper change. Start out with a dime-size amount of salve; use a little more or less as needed.

# Diarrhea

*Diarrhea is often caused by dietary indiscretion; however, it can sometimes occur during illnesses. Typically accompanied by minor abdominal cramping, it tends to clear up once the body has eliminated the offending substance. Because diarrhea can lead to dehydration, be sure to increase your fluid intake. Seek medical aid if your diarrhea is prolonged or frequent, or if blood or mucus is present.*

## Agrimony Tea

Makes 1 cup

Agrimony is a mild astringent that stops irritation in the digestive system, helping to put a stop to diarrhea. It offers a lemony flavor that most people find pleasant. If you are experiencing diarrhea as a flu symptom and also have a sore throat, consider making an extra cup of agrimony tea to use as a soothing gargle.

1 cup boiling water

2 teaspoons dried agrimony

1. Pour the boiling water into a large mug. Add the dried agrimony, cover the mug, and allow the tea to steep for 10 minutes.
2. Relax and drink the tea slowly. Repeat up to four times per day while diarrhea is an issue.

# Catnip-Raspberry Leaf Decoction

Makes 1 quart

Catnip and raspberry leaf are mild astringents that help put a stop to diarrhea. If your diarrhea is accompanied by abdominal cramping, this is a good remedy to try, as raspberry leaves also help smooth muscle tissue to relax. This decoction stays fresh for up to 2 days when refrigerated in a tightly capped container. You can add a little bit of honey if you dislike the natural flavor of the herbs.

8 cups water

2 tablespoons dried catnip

2 tablespoons dried raspberry leaf

1. In a saucepan, combine all the ingredients. Bring the water to a boil over high heat, then reduce the heat to low. Allow the herbs to simmer until the liquid reduces by half.
2. Allow the decoction to cool until it is comfortable to drink.
3. Enjoy a cup warm, or place it in a sealed bottle or jar in the refrigerator to chill.

**Precautions** Never use raspberry leaves that are not completely dried, as fresh ones can cause nausea. Catnip can cause deep relaxation; do not drive or operate machinery until you know how it affects you.

# Dry Skin

*Dehydration, hot or cool indoor air, and long hot showers are just a few things that can contribute to dry skin. Frequent moisturizing can help, as can humidifiers and treatments that call for soothing herbs.*

## Chickweed-Aloe Gel

Makes about ½ cup

Chickweed and aloe vera nourish the skin and infuse it with moisture. This gel absorbs quickly and leaves no odor behind. When refrigerated, it will stay fresh for up to 2 weeks.

½ cup water

¼ cup dried chickweed

¼ cup aloe vera gel

1. In a saucepan, combine the water and chickweed. Bring the mixture to a boil over high heat, then reduce the heat to low. Simmer the mixture until it reduces by half, then remove it from the heat and allow it to cool completely.
2. Dampen a piece of cheesecloth and drape it over the mouth of a funnel. Pour the mixture through the funnel into a glass bowl. Squeeze the liquid from the herbs, wringing the cheesecloth until no more liquid comes out.
3. Add the aloe vera gel to the liquid and use a whisk to blend. Transfer the finished gel to a clean BPA-free squeeze bottle. Cap it tightly and store it in the refrigerator.
4. With your fingertips, apply a thin layer to all affected areas twice per day. Start with a dime-size amount and use more or less next time depending on the size of your skin's dry area.

# Calendula-Comfrey Body Butter

Makes about 2½ cups

Soothing calendula and comfrey offer anti-inflammatory properties that help heal compromised skin, while rich emollients lock moisture in. Use your favorite essential oils to scent it if you like. When stored in a cool, dark place, it stays fresh for up to a year.

½ cup cocoa butter

½ cup coconut oil

½ cup jojoba oil

½ cup shea butter

2 ounces dried calendula

2 ounces dried comfrey

1. In a slow cooker, combine all the ingredients. Select the lowest heat setting, cover the slow cooker, and allow the herbs to steep for 3 to 5 hours. Turn off the heat and allow the infused oil to cool.
2. Drape a piece of cheesecloth over a large mixing bowl. Pour in the infused oil, then wring and twist the cheesecloth until no more oil comes out. Discard the cheesecloth and spent herbs.
3. Place the bowl in the refrigerator and let the mixture cool for about an hour or until it is beginning to firm up.
4. With a hand mixer or immersion blender, whip the body butter for 10 minutes, or until it has a light, fluffy consistency. Return the bowl to the refrigerator for 15 minutes, then transfer the body butter to clean, dry jars with tight-fitting lids.
5. With your fingers, apply a dime-size amount to areas of dry skin. Use a little more or less as needed, and repeat daily for soft, silky skin.

# Earache

*An earache happens when the sensory nerve endings located in the eardrum respond to pressure. Use herbal remedies at the first sign of discomfort. See your doctor if pain worsens or persists, as a severe ear infection can spread or cause permanent hearing impairment.*

## Blue Vervain Infusion and Poultice

Makes 1 treatment

Blue vervain helps relieve pain and increase circulation. This treatment works two ways; the warm poultice soothes the ear area directly from the outside, and the infusion, when drunk, eases the throat pain that can accompany an earache. The infusion has a bitter taste, so you may want to add sweetener to mask it.

2 teaspoons dried blue vervain

1 cup boiling water

1. Put the blue vervain in a tea infuser inside a mug, then add the boiling water. Allow the infusion to steep for 10 minutes.
2. Remove the infuser from the water and allow it to cool until it is still hot but comfortable enough to handle. Transfer the blue vervain to a piece of cheesecloth and fold the cloth into a 4-inch square.
3. Press the poultice against your ear while sipping the tea slowly. You can reactivate the poultice for a second use by wrapping it in a moist towel and microwaving it for 5 to 10 seconds.
4. Repeat the treatment up to three times per day until your earache is gone.

**Precautions** Do not use blue vervain if you are pregnant.

# Garlic-Mullein Infused Oil

## Makes 2 tablespoons

Garlic and mullein flowers offer strong antibacterial and anti-inflammatory properties that can help clear up an earache quickly. This oil will last up to a year when kept in a cool, dark place.

2 tablespoons light olive oil

2 teaspoons crushed or finely chopped dried or freeze-dried garlic

2 teaspoons dried mullein flowers

1. Bring an inch or so of water to a simmer in the base of a double boiler. Reduce the heat to low.

2. In a glass measuring cup, combine the olive oil, garlic, and mullein flowers. Place the measuring cup in the upper part of the double boiler and allow the herbs to steep in the oil for 3 to 5 hours. Turn off the heat and allow the infused oil to cool.

3. Drape a piece of cheesecloth over a small bowl. Pour in the infused oil, then wring and twist the cheesecloth until no more oil comes out. Discard the cheesecloth and spent herbs.

4. Pour the infused oil into a dry, sterilized bottle with a dropper top and allow it to cool completely before capping.

5. With the dropper top, drip 2 to 3 drops into the ear. Place a cotton ball in the ear and leave it in place for 15 minutes. Repeat two or three times per day until the earache is gone.

**Precautions** Garlic may cause a skin rash in sensitive individuals; discontinue if irritation occurs.

# Eczema

*Also known as atopic dermatitis, eczema is characterized by itchy patches of thick, red, scaly skin. This allergic skin condition tends to come and go, and it has a tendency to appear at the same time as seasonal or dietary allergy symptoms.*

## Calendula-Goldenseal Spray

### Makes 1 cup

Calendula and goldenseal impart antiseptic and anti-inflammatory benefits, while witch hazel relieves redness, itching, and scaling. This spray stays fresh for up to a year when kept in a cool, dark place.

1 ounce dried calendula

1 ounce dried goldenseal root

¼ cup jojoba oil

¾ cup witch hazel

1. In a slow cooker, combine the calendula, goldenseal, and jojoba oil. Select the lowest heat setting, cover the slow cooker, and allow the herbs to steep in the oil for 3 to 5 hours. Turn off the heat and allow the infused oil to cool.
2. Drape a piece of cheesecloth over a bowl. Pour in the infused oil, then wring the cheesecloth until no more oil comes out. Discard the spent herbs.
3. Combine the infused oil and the witch hazel in a dark-colored glass bottle with a spray top. Shake gently.
4. Apply 1 or 2 spritzes to the eczema. Massage the spray in, and allow it to absorb. Repeat two or three times per day until the eczema fades.

**Precautions** Omit the goldenseal if you are pregnant or breastfeeding or have high blood pressure.

# Comfrey Salve

Makes about 1 cup

Comfrey has a soothing effect on irritated, itchy skin. It also helps soften rough areas and prevent cracking. Since comfrey stimulates cell regeneration, it speeds the healing process and can help repair damage caused by eczema. This salve lasts up to a year when stored in a cool, dark place.

2 ounces dried comfrey

1 cup light olive oil

1 ounce beeswax

20 drops vitamin E oil

1. In a slow cooker, combine the comfrey and olive oil. Select the lowest heat setting, cover the slow cooker, and allow the herbs to steep in the oil for 3 to 5 hours. Turn off the heat and allow the infused oil to cool.
2. Bring an inch or so of water to a simmer in the base of a double boiler. Reduce the heat to low.
3. Drape a piece of cheesecloth over the upper part of the double boiler. Pour in the infused oil, wringing the cheesecloth until no more oil comes out. Discard the cheesecloth and spent herbs.
4. Add the beeswax to the infused oil and place the double boiler on the base. Gently warm over low heat. When the beeswax melts completely, remove the pan from the heat. Allow the blend to cool slightly, then use a whisk to stir in the vitamin E oil. Quickly pour the salve into clean, dry jars or tins and allow it to cool completely before capping.
5. Apply a pea-size amount to areas of eczema, using a little more or less as needed. Repeat two or three times per day until the eczema fades.

# Fatigue

*The demands of work, school, or raising a family can leave you feeling completely drained. Even a fun-filled vacation can cause fatigue that zaps your strength. Herbs support you far more gently than harsh, caffeinated drinks or sugary snacks do. Try any of these solutions next time you feel like you've hit the wall.*

## Feverfew Tincture

Makes about 2 cups

Feverfew can eliminate the stress and anxiety that often accompany fatigue, and stop associated body aches and headaches as well. This tincture will retain its potency for up to 7 years when kept in a cool, dark place.

8 ounces feverfew

2 cups unflavored 80-proof vodka

1. Put the feverfew in a sterilized pint jar. Add the vodka, filling the jar to the very top and covering the herbs completely.
2. Cap the jar tightly and shake it up. Store it in a cool, dark cabinet and shake it several times a week for 6 to 8 weeks. If any of the alcohol evaporates, add more vodka so that the jar is again full to the top.
3. Dampen a piece of cheesecloth and drape it over the mouth of a funnel. Pour the tincture through the funnel into another sterilized pint jar. Wring the liquid from the feverfew. Discard the spent herbs and transfer the finished tincture to dark-colored glass bottles.
4. Mix 10 drops of tincture into a glass of water or juice and drink it two or three times per day while fatigue is an issue.

**Precautions** Do not use feverfew if you are pregnant or if you are allergic to plants in the ragweed family.

# Licorice-Rosemary Syrup

Makes about 2 cups

Licorice supports adrenal gland health and can help increase energy, while rosemary is an excellent tonic for battling fatigue. Honey is also a natural energy booster that brings a variety of health benefits with it. The syrup will remain fresh for up to 6 months when kept in the refrigerator. If you don't have time to make it, you can get similar benefits by taking a licorice extract supplement and diffusing rosemary essential oil in the area where you spend the most time.

1 ounce dried licorice root, chopped

1 ounce dried rosemary leaves, chopped

2 cups water

1 cup honey

1. In a saucepan, combine the herbs and water. Bring the liquid to a simmer over low heat, cover partially with a lid, and reduce the liquid by half.
2. Transfer the contents of the saucepan to a glass measuring cup, then pour the mixture through a dampened piece of cheesecloth back into the saucepan, wringing the cheesecloth until no more liquid comes out.
3. Add the honey and warm the mixture over low heat, stirring constantly and stopping when the temperature reaches 105°F to 110°F.
4. Pour the syrup into a sterilized jar or bottle and store it in the refrigerator.
5. Take 1 tablespoon orally three times per day until your symptoms subside.

**Precautions** Do not take licorice root if you have high blood pressure, diabetes, kidney problems, or heart disease. Do not use rosemary if you have epilepsy.

# Fever

*Fever is the body's natural defense against infection, so give your system the opportunity to fight if possible. If your fever increases or fails to break, febrifuge (fever-reducing) herbs can help. Be extra-vigilant about seeking medical aid if you have a feverish child. Babies younger than 4 months old need emergency treatment for any fever of 100.4°F or above. Older children should be seen immediately for a fever of 104°F or higher.*

## Feverfew Syrup

Makes about 2 cups

Feverfew gets its name from its ability to act as an effective febrifuge. This syrup is gentle and palatable enough for children to take, and will stay fresh for up to 6 months when refrigerated.

2 ounces dried feverfew

2 cups water

1 cup honey

1. In a saucepan, combine the feverfew and water. Bring the liquid to a simmer over low heat, cover partially with a lid, and reduce the liquid by half.
2. Transfer the contents of the saucepan to a glass measuring cup, then pour the mixture through a dampened piece of cheesecloth back into the saucepan, wringing the liquid from the cheesecloth.
3. Add the honey and warm the mixture over low heat, stirring constantly and stopping when the temperature reaches 105°F to 110°F.
4. Pour the syrup into a sterilized jar or bottle and store it in the refrigerator.
5. Take 1 tablespoon orally three times per day until your symptoms subside. Children under age 12 should take 1 teaspoon three times per day.

**Precautions** Do not take feverfew if you are pregnant or allergic to ragweed.

# Blue Vervain-Raspberry Leaf Tincture

Makes about 2 cups

Blue vervain and raspberry leaf are effective febrifuges that gently reduce fever. This tincture will remain fresh for up to 6 years when stored in a cool, dark place.

4 ounces dried blue vervain

4 ounces dried raspberry leaf

2 cups unflavored 80-proof vodka

1. In a sterilized pint jar, combine the herbs. Add the vodka, filling the jar to the very top and covering the herbs completely.
2. Cap the jar tightly and shake it up. Store it in a cool, dark cabinet and shake it several times per week for 6 to 8 weeks. If any of the alcohol evaporates, add more vodka so that the jar is again full to the top.
3. Dampen a piece of cheesecloth and drape it over the mouth of a funnel. Pour the tincture through the funnel into another sterilized pint jar. Squeeze the liquid from the herbs, wringing the cheesecloth until no more liquid comes out. Discard the roots and transfer the finished tincture to dark-colored glass bottles.
4. Take 10 drops orally two or three times per day. If the taste is too strong for you, you can mix it in a glass of water or juice and drink it.

**Precautions** Do not use blue vervain during pregnancy. Never use raspberry leaves that are not completely dried, as fresh ones can cause nausea.

# Flatulence

*Usually caused by a sudden increase in dietary fiber, flatulence is sometimes physically uncomfortable. More often than not, though, the problem simply involves embarrassment. Herbs help you feel more comfortable and ease the passing of excess intestinal gas.*

## Peppermint-Angelica Tea

Makes 1 cup

Peppermint and angelica promote smooth muscle relaxation, easing tension in the digestive tract and promoting the expulsion of excess gas that causes flatulence.

1 cup boiling water

1 teaspoon dried angelica

1 teaspoon dried peppermint

1. Pour the boiling water into a large mug. Add the dried herbs, cover the mug, and allow the tea to steep for 10 minutes.
2. Relax and drink the tea slowly while inhaling the steam. Repeat up to four times per day.

**Precautions** Omit the angelica if you are pregnant.

# Fresh Ginger-Fennel Decoction

**Makes about 4 cups**

Ginger and fennel aid healthy digestion and help the body get rid of the excess gas that causes flatulence. This tasty decoction makes a nice daily drink, and keeps for up to a week when refrigerated. If you enjoy it, double or triple the recipe to save effort.

8 cups water

1 teaspoon crushed fennel seeds

1 tablespoon minced fresh ginger

Honey or stevia (optional)

1. In a saucepan, combine the water, fennel, and ginger. Turn the heat to high and allow the blend to come to a boil. Reduce the heat to low and let the liquid simmer until it is reduced by half.
2. Allow the decoction to cool. Sweeten it with honey or stevia if you like, then place it in the refrigerator. Drink one cup each evening after dinner. Continue use as long as flatulence is a problem.

**Precautions** Do not use ginger if you take prescription blood thinners, have gallbladder disease, or have a bleeding disorder.

# Flu

*With symptoms that often mimic those of the common cold, influenza is caused by a virus that mutates frequently. It's a good idea to get a yearly flu shot, especially if you work around people who are sick, or if you fall into an at-risk category. If you do end up with the flu, herbs can help ease your symptoms and speed your recovery.*

## Catnip-Hyssop Tea

Makes 1 cup

Catnip and hyssop fight inflammation and ease symptoms, including sore throat and body ache. They also strengthen your immune system, aiding in the fight against the flu virus. This tea is very relaxing, and is ideal for drinking before a nap or bedtime.

1 cup boiling water

1 teaspoon dried catnip

1 teaspoon dried hyssop

1. Pour the boiling water into a large mug. Add the dried herbs, cover the mug, and allow the tea to steep for 10 minutes.
2. Relax and drink the tea slowly while inhaling the steam. Repeat up to four times per day.

**Precautions** Do not use hyssop or catnip during pregnancy. Omit the hyssop if you have epilepsy.

# Garlic, Echinacea, and Goldenseal Syrup

Makes 2 cups

Garlic, echinacea, and goldenseal are potent antiviral herbs that help your body fight the flu naturally. This syrup has a pungent taste despite the honey; you may find it more palatable if you take it with a teaspoon of lemon juice. When kept refrigerated, it remains fresh for up to 6 months.

1 ounce dried or freeze-dried garlic, chopped

1 ounce dried echinacea root, chopped

1 ounce dried goldenseal root, chopped

2 cups water

1 cup honey

1. In a saucepan, combine the herbs and water. Bring the liquid to a simmer over low heat, cover partially with a lid, and reduce the liquid by half.
2. Transfer the contents of the saucepan to a glass measuring cup, then pour the mixture through a dampened piece of cheesecloth back into the saucepan, wringing the cheesecloth until no more liquid comes out.
3. Add the honey and warm the mixture over low heat, stirring constantly and stopping when the temperature reaches 105°F to 110°F.
4. Pour the syrup into a sterilized jar or bottle and store it in the refrigerator.
5. Take 1 tablespoon orally three times per day until your symptoms subside. Children under age 12 should take 1 teaspoon three times per day.

---

**Precautions** Do not use echinacea if you are allergic to ragweed or have an autoimmune disease. Do not use goldenseal if you are pregnant or breastfeeding, or have high blood pressure.

# Gingivitis

*You can develop gingivitis even if you brush your teeth regularly. This common dental disease brings receding gums with it and, over time, can result in loose teeth. Get in the habit of flossing regularly and see your dentist for a cleaning twice a year. Herbs help keep your teeth and gums healthy between professional cleanings.*

## Calendula-Chamomile Mouth Rinse

**Makes 2 cups**

Calendula and chamomile ease inflammation while fighting infection. This mouth rinse has a pleasant floral flavor, and helps sore gums feel better while healing compromised tissue. This rinse will stay fresh for up to a week when stored in the refrigerator.

1 ounce dried calendula

1 ounce dried chamomile

4 cups water

1. In a saucepan, combine the herbs and water. Bring the liquid to a simmer over low heat, cover partially with a lid, and reduce the liquid by half.
2. Transfer the contents of the saucepan to a glass measuring cup, then pour the mixture through a dampened piece of cheesecloth back into the saucepan, wringing the cheesecloth until no more liquid comes out.
3. Transfer the mouth rinse to a clean jar or bottle and store it in the refrigerator.
4. Swish with 2 tablespoons twice per day until your symptoms subside. Do not swallow; spit the rinse into the sink when done. Children under age 12 should use 1 tablespoon twice per day.

**Precautions** Do not use if you are allergic to plants in the ragweed family.

# Goldenseal-Sage Oil Pull

Makes 24 treatments

Goldenseal, sage, and coconut oil combine in this recipe, creating a powerful anti-inflammatory treatment that also helps sore gums heal. If you are new to oil pulling, start gradually and work your way up to the full 15-minute treatment. This blend will stay fresh for up to 6 months when kept in a cool, dark place.

1 ounce dried goldenseal root, chopped

1 ounce dried sage, crumbled

½ cup coconut oil

1. In a slow cooker, combine the herbs and coconut oil. Select the lowest heat setting, cover the slow cooker, and allow the herbs to steep in the oil for 3 to 5 hours. Turn off the heat and allow the infused oil to cool.
2. Drape a piece of cheesecloth over a bowl. Pour in the infused oil, then wring and twist the cheesecloth until no more oil comes out. Discard the cheesecloth and spent herbs.
3. Transfer the infused coconut oil to a clean, dry jar and allow it to cool completely before capping.
4. Take 1 teaspoon of the oil pulling solution and allow it to melt in your mouth. Swish it around and between your teeth, but do not swallow. Keep the solution in your mouth for up to 15 minutes at a time, using a larger amount if you need to.
5. When you are finished, spit the oil into a paper towel and discard it in the trash. Do not spit oil down the sink since this can clog plumbing.

**Precautions** Do not use goldenseal if you are pregnant or breastfeeding, or have high blood pressure.

# Hair Loss

*While hair loss is often viewed as an ailment that affects men, women can experience it as well. There are many causes of thinning hair: Overstyling, stress, and even vitamin imbalances can be to blame. Herbs don't normally help if your hair loss is genetic, but they may stimulate hair growth in many other instances.*

## Ginger Scalp Treatment

Makes ½ cup

Ginger increases circulation in the scalp, stimulating the hair follicles. This treatment will stay fresh for up to 2 months when kept in the refrigerator.

2 ounces fresh gingerroot, chopped

¼ cup sesame oil

1. In a slow cooker, combine the ginger and sesame oil. Select the lowest heat setting, cover the slow cooker, and allow the herbs to steep in the oil for 3 to 5 hours. Turn off the heat and allow the infused oil to cool.
2. Drape a piece of cheesecloth over a bowl. Pour in the infused oil, then wring the cheesecloth until no more oil comes out. Discard the spent ginger.
3. Transfer the infused sesame oil to a clean, dry bottle or jar and allow it to cool completely before capping.
4. Apply 1 tablespoon to the scalp before shampooing your hair. Massage it in.
5. Leave the treatment in place for 30 minutes, then shampoo and condition your hair as usual. Repeat three to four times per week.

**Precautions** Do not use ginger if you take prescription blood thinners, have gallbladder disease, or have a bleeding disorder.

# Ginkgo-Rosemary Tonic

**Makes about 1 cup**

Ginkgo and rosemary combine with witch hazel to increase circulation in the scalp, stimulating your hair follicles. Rosemary adds shine and strength to remaining hair, helping improve your appearance and your self-esteem. This tonic will stay fresh for up to 6 months when refrigerated.

½ ounce dried ginkgo biloba

½ ounce dried rosemary leaves

2 tablespoons fractionated coconut oil

1 cup witch hazel

1. In a slow cooker, combine the herbs and fractionated coconut oil. Select the lowest heat setting, cover the slow cooker, and allow the herbs to steep in the oil for 3 to 5 hours. Turn off the heat and allow the infused oil to cool.
2. Drape a piece of cheesecloth over a bowl. Pour in the infused oil, then wring and twist the cheesecloth until no more oil comes out. Discard the cheesecloth and spent herbs.
3. In a dark-colored glass bottle with a spray top, combine the witch hazel with the infused oil. Shake gently to blend completely.
4. After washing and conditioning your hair, apply a light mist of 1 or 2 spritzes to areas where hair loss is a concern, using a little more if needed. Massage the scalp with your fingertips. Repeat once or twice per day.

**Precautions** Do not use ginkgo biloba if you are taking a monoamine oxidase inhibitor (MAOI) for depression. Ginkgo biloba enhances the effect of blood thinners; talk to your doctor before use. Do not use rosemary if you have epilepsy.

# Halitosis

*Bad breath is unpleasant and embarrassing. Luckily, it's also very easy to treat. Start by staying hydrated, since a dry mouth is the perfect environment for bacterial growth. Practice good oral hygiene, too: Be extra vigilant about brushing and flossing. If herbs don't help, talk to your doctor. Persistent halitosis can be indicative of an underlying medical condition.*

## Peppermint-Sage Mouthwash

### Makes about 2 cups

Peppermint and sage freshen your breath, while the alcohol in this mouthwash kills germs. When made with vodka and kept in a cool, dark place, the rinse will stay fresh for up to 6 years.

6 ounces dried peppermint

2 ounces dried sage

2 cups unflavored 80-proof vodka

1. In a sterilized pint jar, combine the herbs. Add the vodka, filling the jar to the very top and covering the herbs completely.
2. Cap the jar tightly and shake it up. Store it in a cool, dark cabinet and shake it several times per week for 6 to 8 weeks. If any of the alcohol evaporates, add more vodka to fill the jar.
3. Dampen a piece of cheesecloth and drape it over the mouth of a funnel. Pour the tincture through the funnel into another sterilized pint jar. Wring the liquid from the herbs. Discard the spent herbs and transfer the finished tincture to dark-colored glass bottles.
4. After brushing your teeth, swish with 1 tablespoon of mouthwash. Repeat at least twice per day, and more often if you prefer.

# Ginger-Mint Gunpowder Green Tea

**Makes about 30 servings.**

Combined with lemon and spearmint, polyphenols—antioxidants found in gunpowder green tea—help destroy naturally occurring compounds associated with halitosis, tooth decay, and even mouth cancer.

2 lemons

1 (4-inch) piece gingerroot

2 bunches spearmint

1 cup gunpowder green tea leaves

1 cup boiling water

1. Peel the lemons, remove the pith, and cut the rinds into very thin slivers. Place the rinds on a metal rack. (You can juice the lemons for another use.)
2. Peel the gingerroot and cut it into very thin slices; place on the rack with the lemon rinds.
3. Remove the leaves from the spearmint stems, being careful to ensure the leaves remain intact. Discard the stems and place the whole spearmint leaves on the rack with the lemon rinds and gingerroot.
4. Let the lemon rinds, gingerroot, and spearmint leaves dry at room temperature until completely dry and brittle, about 24 hours. Make sure there is no moisture remaining. Crumble the spearmint leaves into small pieces.
5. In a large bowl, mix the lemon rinds, ginger, spearmint leaves, and tea leaves. When they are thoroughly mixed, spoon the mixture into an airtight jar. Store at room temperature for up to a month.
6. To make the tea, pour the boiling water into a large mug. Add 2 teaspoons of the tea mixture, cover the mug, and allow the tea to steep for 10 minutes. Drink the tea.

# Hangover

*Overindulgence happens, but that doesn't mean you have to ride out the aftermath in complete discomfort. Try remedies that address each of your concerns—headache, nausea, and fatigue—while using other remedies to support the detoxification process.*

## Feverfew-Hops Tea

Makes 1 cup

Feverfew addresses your headache, while hops help you relax. This tea is potent enough to help you drop off to sleep so that your body can recover a little bit faster.

1 cup boiling water

1 teaspoon dried feverfew

1 teaspoon dried hops

1. Pour the boiling water into a large mug. Add the dried herbs, cover the mug, and allow the tea to steep for 10 minutes.
2. Relax and drink the tea slowly. Repeat up to three times per day.

**Precautions** Do not use feverfew if you are pregnant or allergic to ragweed.

# Milk Thistle Tincture

**Makes about 2 cups**

Milk thistle supports the liver as it detoxifies the body. This remedy won't help you feel better immediately, but it will make things easier on your system. When stored in a cool, dark place, it will remain fresh for up to 6 years.

8 ounces dried milk thistle

2 cups unflavored 80-proof vodka

1. Put the milk thistle in a sterilized pint jar. Add the vodka, filling the jar to the very top and covering the herbs completely.
2. Cap the jar tightly and shake it up. Store it in a cool, dark cabinet and shake it several times per week for 6 to 8 weeks. If any of the alcohol evaporates, add more vodka so that the jar is again full to the top.
3. Dampen a piece of cheesecloth and drape it over the mouth of a funnel. Pour the tincture through the funnel into another sterilized pint jar. Squeeze the liquid from the herbs, wringing the cheesecloth until no more liquid comes out. Discard the spent herbs and transfer the finished tincture to dark-colored glass bottles.
4. Take 10 drops orally two or three times per day for 7 to 10 days after overindulging. If the taste is too strong for you, you can mix it into a glass of water or juice and drink it. If you are avoiding alcohol, add the tincture to a cup of tea made with boiling water. The alcohol will evaporate within about 5 minutes.

**Precautions** Overuse of milk thistle can cause mild diarrhea. Reduce the amount or frequency if this occurs.

# Headache

*Often caused by stress or muscle tension, headaches are also associated with caffeine withdrawal, eyestrain, and high blood pressure. See your doctor if headaches are frequent or persistent, since they can be symptomatic of an underlying health condition.*

## Blue Vervain-Catnip Tea

Makes 1 cup

Blue vervain and catnip come together to increase circulation and promote relaxation, plus they help ease tension. This blend is ideal for stress headaches.

1 cup boiling water

1 teaspoon dried blue vervain

1 teaspoon dried catnip

1. Pour the boiling water into a large mug. Add the dried herbs, cover the mug, and allow the tea to steep for 10 minutes.
2. Relax and drink the tea slowly. Repeat up to three times per day.

**Precautions** Do not use blue vervain or catnip during pregnancy.

# Skullcap Tincture

Makes about 2 cups

Skullcap is a mild sedative that has a beneficial effect on nerve pain. If you get migraines and can't take feverfew, skullcap is an alternative worth considering. This tincture provides quick relief. Skullcap can also be found in a convenient capsule form if you would prefer that. When kept in a cool, dark place, this tincture retains freshness for up to 6 years.

8 ounces skullcap

2 cups unflavored 80-proof vodka

1. Put the skullcap in a sterilized pint jar. Add the vodka, filling the jar to the very top and covering the herbs completely.
2. Cap the jar tightly and shake it up. Store it in a cool, dark cabinet and shake it several times per week for 6 to 8 weeks. If any of the alcohol evaporates, add more vodka so that the jar is again full to the top.
3. Dampen a piece of cheesecloth and drape it over the mouth of a funnel. Pour the tincture through the funnel into another sterilized pint jar. Squeeze the liquid from the herbs, wringing the cheesecloth until no more liquid comes out. Discard the spent herbs and transfer the finished tincture to dark-colored glass bottles.
4. Take 1 teaspoon orally two or three times per day when you have a headache. If the taste is too strong for you, you can mix it into a glass of water or juice and drink it.

**Precautions** Do not take skullcap during pregnancy.

# Heartburn

*The searing pain of heartburn is a symptom of gastroesophageal reflux disease (GERD), a digestive disease occurring when stomach acid moves into the esophagus. GERD may be caused by increased acid production, obesity, overeating, tight clothing, and a number of other factors. If you are pregnant, your heartburn could be happening as your growing baby places increased pressure on your stomach. Herbs won't cure your heartburn, but they can bring relief while you sort out the underlying cause.*

## Fresh Ginger Tea

Makes 1 cup

Ginger improves blood flow throughout the body and can help you get over heartburn faster. Its anti-inflammatory and pain-relieving capacities soothe your esophagus, which becomes irritated when it is exposed to stomach acid.

1 cup boiling water

1 tablespoon chopped fresh gingerroot

1. Pour the boiling water into a large mug. Add the ginger, cover the mug, and allow the tea to steep for 10 minutes.
2. Relax and drink the tea slowly while inhaling the steam. Repeat up to four times per day whenever heartburn is an issue.

**Precautions** Do not use ginger if you take prescription blood thinners, have gallbladder disease, or have a bleeding disorder.

# Fennel-Angelica Syrup

Makes 2 cups

Fennel and angelica improve blood flow throughout the digestive tract and offer soothing comfort to an irritated esophagus while helping speed up digestion. This syrup will stay fresh for up to 6 months in the refrigerator.

1 ounce dried angelica

1 tablespoon fennel seeds

2 cups water

1 cup honey

1. In a saucepan, combine the herbs and water. Bring the liquid to a simmer over low heat, cover partially with a lid, and reduce the liquid by half.
2. Transfer the contents of the saucepan to a glass measuring cup, then pour the mixture through a dampened piece of cheesecloth back into the saucepan, wringing the cheesecloth until no more liquid comes out.
3. Add the honey and warm the mixture over low heat, stirring constantly and stopping when the temperature reaches 105°F to 110°F.
4. Pour the syrup into a sterilized jar or bottle and store it in the refrigerator.
5. Take 1 tablespoon orally three times per day until your heartburn symptoms subside.

# Hemorrhoids

*Hemorrhoids are distended veins in the rectum and around the anus. When they are inflamed, they cause bleeding, intense itching, and pain. Usually caused by prolonged sitting or straining during bowel movements, hemorrhoids commonly occur during pregnancy. Anti-inflammatory herbs provide comfort and help speed healing.*

## Calendula-Witch Hazel Spray

Makes 1 cup

Calendula and witch hazel impart antiseptic and anti-inflammatory benefits. Witch hazel also helps shrink swollen veins and tissue while easing the itch that accompanies hemorrhoids. This spray stays fresh for up to a year when kept in a cool, dark place.

2 ounces dried calendula
¼ cup light olive oil
¾ cup witch hazel

1. In a slow cooker, combine the calendula and olive oil. Select the lowest heat setting, cover the slow cooker, and allow the herbs to steep in the oil for 3 to 5 hours. Turn off the heat and let the infused oil cool.
2. Drape a piece of cheesecloth over a bowl. Pour in the infused oil, then wring the cheesecloth until no more oil comes out. Discard the spent herbs.
3. In a dark glass bottle with a spray top, combine the infused oil and the witch hazel. Shake gently to blend completely.
4. Apply 2 or 3 spritzes to a cotton cosmetic pad and apply it to the affected area. Repeat two or three times per day, especially after bowel movements and before bed. Continue use as long as hemorrhoids are a concern.

# Chickweed-Goldenseal Ointment with St. John's Wort

**Makes about ¼ cup**

Chickweed, goldenseal, and St. John's wort help put a stop to the itching and inflammation that accompany hemorrhoids while soothing the stretched, sensitive skin that covers the veins. This ointment lasts up to a year when stored in a cool, dark place.

1 tablespoon dried chickweed

1 tablespoon chopped dried goldenseal root

1 tablespoon dried St. John's wort

2 tablespoons jojoba oil

1 tablespoon light olive oil

1 tablespoon cocoa butter

1 tablespoon grated beeswax or
    beeswax pastilles

3 drops vitamin E oil

1. In a slow cooker, combine the herbs with the jojoba oil, olive oil, and cocoa butter. Select the lowest heat setting, cover the slow cooker, and allow the herbs to steep for 3 to 5 hours. Turn off the heat and allow the infused oil to cool.

2. Bring an inch or so of water to a simmer in the base of a double boiler. Reduce the heat to low.

3. Drape a piece of cheesecloth over the upper part of the double boiler. Pour in the infused oil, then wring the cheesecloth until no more oil comes out. Discard the cheesecloth and spent herbs.

4. Add the beeswax to the infused oil and place the double boiler on the base. Gently warm over low heat. When the beeswax melts completely, remove the pan from the heat and add the vitamin E oil. Immediately pour the mixture into clean, dry jars or tins and allow it to cool completely before capping.

5. With a cotton cosmetic pad, apply a pea-size amount to the affected area. Repeat after each bowel movement and once more before going to bed. Continue as long as hemorrhoids are a problem.

**Precautions** Do not use goldenseal if you are pregnant or breastfeeding, or if you have high blood pressure.

# High Blood Pressure

*Also known as hypertension, high blood pressure can increase your risk of early cognitive decline, heart disease, kidney failure, and stroke if left untreated. Losing weight, exercising, and meditating are some ways to naturally encourage healing. If you can't bring your blood pressure down on your own within 2 months, see your doctor immediately.*

## Angelica Infusion

Makes 1 quart

Angelica contains compounds that act very much like the calcium channel blockers (drugs that relax and widen blood vessels affecting arterial wall muscles) often prescribed to reduce high blood pressure. This infusion is somewhat bitter, but it can be mixed with a little sweetener or juice if you like. When refrigerated, it will stay fresh for 3 days.

4 teaspoons dried angelica

4 cups boiling water

4 teaspoons fresh lemon juice

1. In a teapot, combine the dried angelica and the boiling water. Cover the pot and allow the infusion to steep for 10 minutes, then add the lemon juice.
2. Relax and drink a cup of the infusion slowly. You can refrigerate the rest and sip it over the course of a few days, either reheated or over ice.

**Precautions** Do not take angelica during pregnancy or if you are taking anticoagulants.

# Dandelion-Lavender Tincture

Makes about 2 cups

Dandelions are an excellent source of potassium, which naturally controls salt levels and helps lower blood pressure. Lavender's scent and oils relax and balance the nervous system.

4 ounces dried dandelion root, finely chopped

4 ounces dried lavender leaves, chopped

2 cups unflavored 80-proof vodka

1. In a sterilized pint jar, combine the herbs. Add the vodka, filling the jar to the very top and covering the herbs completely.
2. Cap the jar tightly and shake it up. Store it in a cool, dark cabinet and shake it several times per week for 6 to 8 weeks. If any of the alcohol evaporates, add more vodka so that the jar is again full to the top.
3. Dampen a piece of cheesecloth and drape it over the mouth of a funnel. Pour the tincture through the funnel into another sterilized pint jar. Squeeze the liquid from the herbs, wringing the cheesecloth until no more liquid comes out. Discard the spent herbs and transfer the finished tincture to dark-colored glass bottles.
4. Take 10 drops orally two or three times per day. If the taste is too strong for you, you can mix it into a glass of water or juice and drink it. Continue while pursuing lifestyle changes and taking positive actions to improve your blood pressure.

**Precautions** Do not use this tincture for longer than 2 months. Excessive use of dandelions can lead to dangerously low blood pressure levels. When taken by mouth, excessive amounts of lavender can lead to constipation, headache, and increased appetite. If you experience any adverse side effects, consult your physician immediately.

# Hives

*Although hives are sometimes associated with severe stress or psychological distress, they typically appear in response to an allergen such as a harsh detergent, dry cleaning chemicals, or even seemingly benign foods such as strawberries.*

## Licorice-Chamomile Spray

Makes 1 cup

Chamomile and licorice root tinctures combine with witch hazel in this simple spray. All three ingredients help ease inflammation and itching, and the witch hazel can help shrink swollen tissue. This spray stays fresh for up to a year in the refrigerator.

¾ cup witch hazel

2 tablespoons chamomile tincture

2 tablespoons licorice root tincture

1. In a dark-colored glass bottle with a spray top, combine all the ingredients. Shake gently to blend completely.
2. Apply 1 or 2 spritzes to each area where hives are a concern. Repeat three or four times per day or even more often if needed. Allow the spray to dry before covering the area with clothing.

**Precautions** Omit the chamomile if you are allergic to ragweed or are taking prescription blood thinners. Omit the licorice if you have high blood pressure, diabetes, kidney problems, or heart disease.

# Rosemary-Comfrey Salve

Makes about 1 cup

Rosemary contains constituents that block histamines. It's an excellent salve for hives associated with contact dermatitis caused by an allergic reaction. This salve lasts for up to a year when stored in a cool, dark place.

1 cup light olive oil

1 ounce dried rosemary, crumbled

1 ounce dried comfrey

1 ounce beeswax

1. In a slow cooker, combine the olive oil, rosemary, and comfrey. Select the lowest heat setting, cover the slow cooker, and allow the herbs to steep in the oil for 3 to 5 hours. Turn off the heat and allow the infused oil to cool.

2. Bring an inch or so of water to a simmer in the base of a double boiler. Reduce the heat to low.

3. Drape a piece of cheesecloth over the upper part of the double boiler. Pour in the infused oil, then wring and twist the cheesecloth until no more oil comes out. Discard the cheesecloth and spent herbs.

4. Add the beeswax to the infused oil and place the double boiler on the base. Gently warm over low heat. When the beeswax melts completely, remove the blend from the heat. Quickly pour the salve into clean, dry jars or tins and allow it to cool completely before capping.

5. With a cotton cosmetic pad or your fingertips, apply a dime-size amount to each area where hives are a concern, using a little more or less as needed. Repeat three to four times per day until the hives are gone.

# Indigestion

*Bloating, belching, and discomfort are signs that you've eaten something that didn't agree with you, or that you've perhaps eaten a bit too much of a favorite food. Herbs can bring quick relief without any of the side effects that can accompany commercial antacids.*

## Chamomile-Angelica Tea

Makes 1 cup

Angelica and chamomile relax the muscles in the gastrointestinal tract while helping improve circulation and keep things moving. A teaspoon of honey and a squeeze of fresh lemon will make the tea go down a bit more easily.

1 cup boiling water

1 teaspoon dried angelica

1 teaspoon dried chamomile

1. Pour the boiling water into a large mug. Add the dried herbs, cover the mug, and allow the tea to steep for 10 minutes.
2. Relax and drink the tea slowly. Repeat up to four times per day.

**Precautions** Do not use angelica during pregnancy. Do not take chamomile if you are allergic to plants in the ragweed family.

# Ginger Syrup

Makes 2 cups

Ginger soothes the digestive tract and improves blood flow, helping you digest food more easily. Take this remedy with a teaspoon of fresh lemon juice for even faster relief. This syrup will stay fresh for up to 6 months in the refrigerator.

2 ounces fresh gingerroot, chopped

2 cups water

1 cup honey

1. In a saucepan, combine the ginger and water. Bring the liquid to a simmer over low heat, cover partially with a lid, and reduce the liquid by half.
2. Transfer the contents of the saucepan to a glass measuring cup, then pour the mixture through a dampened piece of cheesecloth back into the saucepan, wringing the cheesecloth until no more liquid comes out.
3. Add the honey and warm the mixture over low heat, stirring constantly and stopping when the temperature reaches 105°F to 110°F.
4. Pour the syrup into a sterilized jar or bottle and store it in the refrigerator.
5. Take 1 tablespoon orally three or four times per day until your symptoms subside. Children under age 12 should take 1 teaspoon up to three times per day.

**Precautions** Do not use ginger if you take prescription blood thinners, have gallbladder disease, or have a bleeding disorder.

# Insect Bites

*Mosquitos, chiggers, biting gnats, and fleas are just some of the pests that leave raised, red bites behind. Sometimes so itchy that they leave you unable to focus or sleep, these little bites are readily soothed with simple plant-based remedies.*

## Fresh Basil-Mullein Salve

Makes 1 treatment

Basil and mullein offer anti-inflammatory benefits, and basil contains a constituent called eugenol, which helps numb the itch. The honey in this remedy binds the herbs to your skin and helps your bug bites heal faster. If you have lots of insect bites or your whole family is affected, you can easily double or triple the recipe so that there's enough to go around. When kept in the refrigerator, it stays fresh for up to 2 days.

1 tablespoon fresh basil
1 tablespoon fresh mullein
1 tablespoon raw honey

1. In a mini food processer, combine all the ingredients. Process until blended into a fine paste.
2. With your fingertip or a cotton swab, apply a drop or two of the blend to each of your insect bites.
3. Place any leftover salve in a small container with a tight-fitting lid and refrigerate for later use. Repeat the treatment as often as itching recurs.

# Peppermint-Plantain Balm

**Makes about 5 tablespoons
(enough to fill 5 lip balm tubes)**

If you spend lots of time in buggy environments, you'll find that these tubes of insect bite balm are both convenient and easy to use. The peppermint and plantain soothe the itch while helping your skin heal faster, and as a bonus, you can use the balm to keep your lips feeling soft and smooth. This remedy lasts for up to a year when stored in a cool, dark place.

1 tablespoon dried peppermint

1 tablespoon dried plantain

2 tablespoons jojoba oil

1 tablespoon light olive oil

1 tablespoon cocoa butter

4 teaspoons grated beeswax or
   beeswax pastilles

3 drops vitamin E oil

20 drops peppermint essential oil (optional)

1. In a slow cooker, combine the herbs with the jojoba oil, olive oil, and cocoa butter. Select the lowest heat setting, cover the slow cooker, and allow the herbs to steep in the oil for 3 to 5 hours. Turn off the heat and allow the infused oil to cool.

2. Bring an inch or so of water to a simmer in the base of a double boiler. Reduce the heat to low.

3. Drape a piece of cheesecloth over the upper part of the double boiler. Pour in the infused oil, then wring and twist the cheesecloth until no more oil comes out. Discard the cheesecloth and spent herbs.

4. Add the beeswax to the infused oil and place the double boiler on the base. Remove the pan from the heat as soon as the wax melts, then add the vitamin E oil and peppermint essential oil (if using). Immediately pour the mixture into clean, dry lip balm tubes or tins and allow to cool completely before capping.

5. Apply a dab of balm to each insect bite as often as needed to stop itching.

# Insomnia

*Anxiety, caffeine, and stress are prime contributors to insomnia. Overexposure to electronics, especially during the hour before bedtime, is another major culprit. Be sure to address these factors while using herbal remedies that promote sleep.*

## Valerian Tea with Hops and Passionflower

Makes 1 cup

Valerian, hops, and passionflower combine to create a soothing blend that eases tension and anxiety while promoting deep, restful sleep.

1 cup boiling water

1 teaspoon chopped dried valerian root

½ teaspoon crushed dried hops

½ teaspoon dried passionflower

1. Pour the boiling water into a large mug. Add the dried herbs, cover the mug, and allow the tea to steep for 10 minutes.
2. Relax and drink the tea slowly. Repeat each night before bedtime, during periods of time when insomnia is an issue.

**Precautions** Do not give hops to prepubescent children of either gender. Do not use passionflower if you have prostate problems or baldness. Do not use during pregnancy.

# Chamomile-Catnip Syrup

## Makes 2 cups

While chamomile and catnip are both deeply relaxing herbs, this recipe is mild enough for children to take when occasional sleeplessness keeps them wide awake. This syrup stays fresh for up to 6 months when stored in the refrigerator.

1 ounce dried chamomile

1 ounce dried catnip

2 cups water

1 cup honey

1. In a saucepan, combine the chamomile, catnip, and water. Bring the liquid to a simmer over low heat, cover partially with a lid, and reduce the liquid by half.
2. Transfer the contents of the saucepan to a glass measuring cup, then pour the mixture through a dampened piece of cheesecloth back into the saucepan, wringing the cheesecloth until no more liquid comes out.
3. Add the honey and warm the mixture over low heat, stirring constantly and stopping when the temperature reaches 105°F to 110°F.
4. Pour the syrup into a sterilized jar or bottle and store it in the refrigerator.
5. Take 1 tablespoon orally 30 minutes before bed. Children under age 12 should take 1 teaspoon 30 minutes before bedtime.

**Precautions** Do not use catnip during pregnancy. Do not use chamomile if you are allergic to plants in the ragweed family or if you take prescription blood thinners.

# Jock Itch

*Caused by the tinea fungus and characterized by an itchy, painful rash, jock itch tends to affect the groin, inner thighs, and buttocks area. While its name suggests that this is an ailment that affects only men, it can affect anyone. Be sure to keep the affected area clean and dry, as this will help treatments work faster.*

## Infused Garlic Oil

Makes 1 cup

Garlic is a strong antifungal agent that targets the microbes that cause jock itch. While this oil has a pungent smell, it soothes your irritated skin, helps take away the itch, and kills the fungus.

4 ounces dried or freeze-dried garlic, chopped

1 cup light olive oil

1. In a slow cooker, combine the garlic and olive oil. Select the lowest heat setting, cover the slow cooker, and allow the herbs to steep in the oil for at least 5 hours or overnight. Turn off the heat and allow the infused oil to cool.
2. Drape a cheesecloth over a bowl. Pour in the infused oil, then wring and twist the cheesecloth until no more oil comes out. Discard the cheesecloth and garlic.
3. Pour the infused oil into a dry, sterilized jar or bottle and allow it to cool completely before capping.
4. With a cotton cosmetic pad, apply ¼ teaspoon to each area of concern. Use a new pad for each area that you treat. Repeat three or four times per day and continue use for at least a week after the jock itch fades.

**Precautions** Garlic can cause skin irritation in sensitive individuals. Discontinue use if this occurs.

# Calendula, Chamomile, and Goldenseal Spray

**Makes about 1 cup**

Calendula, chamomile, and goldenseal offer strong antifungal benefits while helping compromised skin heal. The witch hazel that serves as the base for this treatment cools the hot, itchy feel that accompanies jock itch. This spray stays fresh for up to a year in the refrigerator.

1 tablespoon chopped dried goldenseal root

1 tablespoon dried calendula

1 tablespoon dried chamomile

¼ cup fractionated coconut oil

¾ cup witch hazel

1. In a slow cooker, combine the herbs and fractionated coconut oil. Select the lowest heat setting, cover the slow cooker, and allow the herbs to steep in the oil for 3 to 5 hours. Turn off the heat and allow the infused oil to cool.

2. Drape a piece of cheesecloth over a bowl. Pour in the infused oil, then wring and twist the cheesecloth until no more oil comes out. Discard the cheesecloth and spent herbs.

3. In a dark-colored glass bottle with a spray top, combine the infused oil with the witch hazel. Shake gently to blend completely.

4. Apply 1 or 2 spritzes to each area where jock itch is a concern. Repeat three or four times per day or more often if needed. Continue use for at least a week after the jock itch fades.

**Precautions** Omit the goldenseal if you are pregnant or breastfeeding, or have high blood pressure.

# Keratosis Pilaris

*Keratosis pilaris is a common skin condition that occurs when the skin produces too much keratin. With dry, rough patches and pimple-like bumps that often appear on the backs of your arms and thighs, "chicken skin" is harmless but unsightly.*

## Chickweed Scrub

Makes 2 cups

Chickweed and baking soda offer effective but gentle exfoliation, and chickweed helps ease the inflammation that comes with keratosis pilaris. This scrub will stay fresh for up to 6 months when stored in a sealed container in a cool, dry place.

1 cup baking soda

1 cup crushed dried chickweed

1. In a food processer or blender, combine the baking soda and crushed chickweed. Process until a fine powder results.
2. While showering or bathing, combine 1 tablespoon of the scrub with an equal amount of your favorite liquid body wash. Apply the entire amount to areas affected by keratosis pilaris, scrubbing gently while using circular, massaging motions. Repeat at least three times per week.

**Precautions** Baking soda can dry the skin. Spot test this scrub first before beginning repeated use. If you experience dryness or burning of the skin, discontinue immediately.

# Calendula-Chamomile Body Butter

Makes about 2½ cups

Soothing calendula and chamomile offer anti-inflammatory properties that help irritated skin, while rich emollients seal moisture inside. This body butter makes a nice all-over moisturizer, and you can use your favorite essential oils to add your favorite scent. When stored in a cool, dark place, this body butter stays fresh for up to a year.

2 ounces dried calendula

2 ounces dried chamomile

½ cup coconut oil

½ cup jojoba oil

½ cup cocoa butter

½ cup shea butter

1. In a slow cooker, combine all the ingredients. Select the lowest heat setting, cover the slow cooker, and allow the herbs to steep for 3 to 5 hours. Turn off the heat and allow the infused oil to cool.

2. Drape a cheesecloth over a large mixing bowl. Pour in the infused oil, then wring and twist the cheesecloth until no more oil comes out. Discard the cheesecloth and spent herbs.

3. Place the bowl in the refrigerator and let the mixture cool for about 1 hour, or until it begins to firm.

4. With a hand mixer or immersion blender, whip the body butter for 10 minutes, or until it has a light, fluffy consistency. Return the bowl to the refrigerator for 15 minutes, then transfer the body butter to clean, dry jars with tight-fitting lids.

5. With your fingers, apply a dime-size amount to areas where keratosis pilaris is a concern. Use a little more or less as needed, and repeat daily for soft, silky skin.

# Laryngitis

*When your voice box becomes swollen and inflamed from infection, irritation, or overuse, laryngitis is the result. While herbs will soothe discomfort, you should see your doctor if the problem is prolonged, since persistent hoarseness can signify an underlying illness.*

## Mullein-Sage Tea

Makes 1 cup

Mullein and sage ease the pain and irritation of laryngitis while helping compromised tissue heal faster. This soothing remedy has a strong herbal taste; you may want to add a teaspoon of lemon juice or honey to make it go down a bit more easily.

1 cup boiling water

1 teaspoon dried mullein

1 teaspoon dried sage

1. Pour the boiling water into a large mug. Add the dried herbs, cover the mug, and allow the tea to steep for 10 minutes.
2. Relax while drinking the tea. Repeat as often as needed.

# Ginger Gargle

Makes 1 cup

Ginger eases pain and inflammation in your throat, and the honey in this recipe provides a light coating while offering additional anti-inflammatory benefits. If you like, you can use this recipe to make a soothing tea, too.

1 cup boiling water

1 teaspoon minced fresh or dried ginger

1 teaspoon honey

1. Pour the boiling water into a large mug. Add the ginger and honey, cover the mug, and allow the blend to steep for 10 minutes.
2. Let the liquid cool to room temperature or refrigerate it if you prefer a cooler sensation. Gargle with 1 tablespoon at a time, repeating as often as needed to bring relief from throat irritation. Store for up to 3 days in the refrigerator.

**Precautions** Do not use if you take prescription blood thinners, have gallbladder disease, or have a bleeding disorder.

# Menopause

*Menopause is a completely normal change in female hormone function, but it unfortunately often brings physical discomfort with it. In addition to these natural treatments, regular exercise can help, and so can a diet high in non-GMO soy, which is a good source of natural plant estrogen.*

## Fennel-Sage Decoction

**Makes 1 cup**

This fennel and sage decoction offers estrogenic properties, and is a good one for dealing with hot flashes as they arise. You can make a larger batch if you like, and keep it refrigerated for up to a week so that it's on hand when you need it. You can also add a sweetener if you like.

2 cups water

1 teaspoon fennel seeds

1 teaspoon sage

1. In a saucepan, combine all the ingredients and bring to a boil over high heat. Reduce the heat to low and allow the blend to simmer until the liquid is reduced by half.
2. Let the decoction cool for 5 or 10 minutes. Relax while drinking the entire amount.

# Black Cohosh Tincture

Makes about 2 cups

Black cohosh contains isoflavones that mimic female hormonal activity. It is useful for managing the mild depression, vaginal dryness, and hot flashes associated with menopause. This tincture will stay fresh for up to 6 years when kept in a cool, dark place.

8 ounces black cohosh, finely chopped

2 cups unflavored 80-proof vodka

1. Put the black cohosh in a sterilized pint jar. Add the vodka, filling the jar to the very top and covering the herbs completely.
2. Cap the jar tightly and shake it up. Store it in a cool, dark cabinet and shake it several times per week for 6 to 8 weeks. If any of the alcohol evaporates, add more vodka so that the jar is again full to the top.
3. Dampen a piece of cheesecloth and drape it over the mouth of a funnel. Pour the tincture through the funnel into another sterilized pint jar. Squeeze the liquid from the herbs, wringing the cheesecloth until no more liquid comes out. Discard the spent herbs and transfer the finished tincture to dark-colored glass bottles.
4. Take ½ teaspoon orally once per day. If the taste is too strong for you, you can mix the tincture into a glass of water or juice and drink it.

# Mental Focus

*Anxiety, insomnia, illness, and stress are just a few of the things that can rob you of your ability to think clearly. Certain herbs can sharpen your focus and make everyday life easier while you take steps to eliminate the cause of your brain fog.*

## Ginseng-Rosemary Tea

Makes 1 cup

Ginseng offers steady energy while increasing circulation and promoting a sense of alertness; rosemary stimulates the thought process and helps you retain information. If you need an easier way to take your daily dose of ginseng, you can opt for a high-quality supplement.

1 cup boiling water

1 teaspoon dried ginseng

1 teaspoon dried rosemary

1. Pour the boiling water into a large mug. Add the dried herbs, cover the mug, and allow the tea to steep for 10 minutes.
2. Relax and drink the tea slowly. Repeat up to two times per day.

**Precautions** Do not use ginseng if you are pregnant or have high blood pressure. Omit the rosemary if you have epilepsy.

# Ginkgo Biloba Tincture

Makes about 2 cups

Ginkgo biloba increases circulation, oxygenating brain tissue and helping improve cognition. If you don't like the idea of taking a daily tincture, you can opt for a high-quality ginkgo capsule instead. This tincture offers a cost-effective solution and will stay fresh for up to 6 years when stored in a cool, dark place.

8 ounces ginkgo biloba, finely chopped

2 cups unflavored 80-proof vodka

1. Put the ginkgo biloba in a sterilized pint jar. Add the vodka, filling the jar to the very top and covering the herbs completely.
2. Cap the jar tightly and shake it up. Store it in a cool, dark cabinet and shake it several times per week for 6 to 8 weeks. If any of the alcohol evaporates, add more vodka so that the jar is again full to the top.
3. Dampen a piece of cheesecloth and drape it over the mouth of a funnel. Pour the tincture through the funnel into another sterilized pint jar. Squeeze the liquid from the herbs, wringing the cheesecloth until no more liquid comes out. Discard the spent herbs and transfer the finished tincture to dark-colored glass bottles.
4. Take 10 drops orally once per day. If the taste is too strong for you, you can mix it into a glass of water or juice and drink it.

**Precautions** Do not use if taking a monoamine oxidase inhibitor (MAOI) for depression. Ginkgo biloba enhances the effect of blood thinners, so talk to your doctor before use.

# Mental Wellness

*Demanding careers, tight schedules, and events that drain your emotions can leave you anxious, depressed, and lacking energy. Herbs can often make a marked difference, but be sure to follow all safety recommendations and never stop taking a prescription abruptly or without your doctor's knowledge.*

## St. John's Wort Tea

Makes 1 cup

Though simple and straightforward, this remedy is an excellent one for anxiety and minor depression. If tea isn't for you, find a high-quality St. John's wort supplement and take it as directed.

1 cup boiling water

1 teaspoon dried St. John's wort

1. Pour the boiling water into a large mug. Add the St. John's wort, cover the mug, and allow the tea to steep for 10 minutes.
2. Relax and drink the tea slowly while inhaling the steam. Repeat up to two times per day.

**Precautions** Do not take St. John's wort if you take monoamine oxidase inhibitor (MAOI) or selective serotonin reuptake inhibitor (SSRI) pharmaceuticals.

# Chamomile-Passionflower Decoction

Makes 1 cup

Chamomile and passionflower help you deal with stress by promoting relaxation and easing anxiety. This is a very soothing blend that can help you fall asleep faster when worries lead to insomnia. Feel free to add a sweetener if you like.

2 cups water

1 teaspoon dried chamomile

1 teaspoon dried passionflower

1. In a saucepan, combine all the ingredients and bring to a boil over high heat. Reduce the heat to low and allow the blend to simmer until the liquid is reduced by half.
2. Let the decoction cool for 5 to 10 minutes. Relax while drinking the entire amount.

**Precautions** Do not use chamomile if you are allergic to plants in the ragweed family or if you take prescription blood thinners. Do not use passionflower if you are pregnant or if you have baldness or prostate problems.

# Muscle Cramps

*The aching and spasms that come with cramped muscles can prevent you from moving normally, and they can even keep you up at night. Herbs can ease muscle tension and help you rest so your body can heal. If you experience cramps frequently, consult your doctor, as cramps and spasms can be symptomatic of an underlying medical condition.*

## Rosemary Liniment

Makes ½ cup

Rosemary stimulates circulation, plus it contains constituents that relieve pain. This simple remedy is made even more effective when you add rosemary essential oil. Kept in the refrigerator, it will stay fresh for up to 7 years.

2 tablespoons rosemary tincture

⅓ cup unflavored 80-proof vodka

20 drops rosemary essential oil (optional)

1. In a dark-colored glass bottle, combine the ingredients by shaking gently.
2. With a cotton cosmetic pad, apply 5 to 10 drops to the cramped area. Use a little more or less as needed.
3. Repeat hourly while having cramps or muscle spasms.

**Precautions** Do not use rosemary if you have epilepsy.

# Ginger Salve

Makes about 1 cup

Ginger increases blood flow while offering a deeply penetrating warming effect. Its anti-inflammatory and pain-relieving properties make it a simple yet effective choice for dealing with muscle cramps.

2 ounces dry or freeze-dried gingerroot, chopped

1 cup light olive oil

1 ounce beeswax

1. In a slow cooker, combine the ginger and olive oil. Select the lowest heat setting, cover the slow cooker, and allow the ginger to steep in the oil for 3 to 5 hours. Turn off the heat and allow the infused oil to cool.

2. Bring an inch or so of water to a simmer in the base of a double boiler. Reduce the heat to low.

3. Drape a cheesecloth over the upper part of the double boiler. Pour in the infused oil, then wring and twist the cheesecloth until no more oil comes out. Discard the cheesecloth and spent herbs.

4. Add the beeswax to the infused oil and place the double boiler on the base. Gently warm over low heat. When the beeswax melts completely, remove the pan from the heat. Quickly pour the salve into clean, dry jars or tins and allow it to cool completely before capping.

5. With your fingertips, massage a dime-size amount into the cramped area. Use a little more or less as needed, and repeat as often as required when cramping is a problem.

**Precautions** Do not use ginger if you take prescription blood thinners, have gallbladder disease, or have a bleeding disorder.

# Nausea

*Sometimes accompanying an illness such as influenza, nausea can also be caused by a foodborne pathogen. Herbal remedies offer quick relief, allowing you to go about your daily routine more comfortably.*

## Peppermint Decoction

Makes 1 cup

This peppermint decoction offers an uplifting, refreshing aroma that starts to settle your stomach before you even take a sip. Thanks to its antispasmodic benefits, peppermint calms nausea caused by a variety of illnesses. You can add a sweetener if you like.

2 teaspoons peppermint leaves

2 cups water

1. In a saucepan, combine the peppermint and water and bring to a boil over high heat. Reduce the heat to low and allow the blend to simmer until the liquid is reduced by half.
2. Let the decoction cool for 5 to 10 minutes. Relax and breathe deeply while drinking the entire amount. Repeat three or four times per day while recovering, or less often if you're prone to heartburn, since peppermint can exacerbate the problem.

# Chamomile-Ginger Tea

Makes 1 cup

Chamomile and ginger improve circulation while helping the body deal with the imbalances that lead to nausea. This remedy is a simple but effective one for motion sickness as well as for nausea associated with chemotherapy, morning sickness, or gastrointestinal distress.

1 cup boiling water

1 teaspoon dried chamomile

1 teaspoon chopped fresh gingerroot

1. Pour the boiling water into a large mug. Add the chamomile and ginger, cover the mug, and allow the tea to steep for 10 minutes.
2. Relax and drink the tea slowly while inhaling the steam. Repeat up to four times per day.

**Precautions** Do not use ginger if you take prescription blood thinners, have gallbladder disease, or have a bleeding disorder. Do not use chamomile if you are allergic to plants in the ragweed family or if you take prescription blood thinners.

# Oily Skin

*Oily skin is the result of an over-production of sebum, an exocrine secretion used to moisturize and waterproof the skin. Harsh treatments can overdry your skin and encourage even more sebum production, making the problem worse than it was to start with. Treat your oily skin gently, and balance will be far easier to achieve.*

## Rosemary Toner

**Makes about 1 cup**

Rosemary is a gentle astringent that helps balance skin. The witch hazel that serves as the base for this toner refreshes your skin without drying it out. This toner stays fresh for up to 6 months when stored in the refrigerator.

1 cup witch hazel

2 tablespoons rosemary tincture

1. In a dark-colored glass bottle, combine the ingredients by shaking gently.
2. With a cotton cosmetic pad, apply ¼ teaspoon to your face. Use a little more or less as needed.
3. Repeat twice per day or anytime you need to refresh your skin.

**Precautions** Do not use rosemary if you have epilepsy.

# Peppermint Scrub

Makes 1 cup

Peppermint cools and comforts the skin while gently cleansing it. There are no harsh detergents in this recipe, and it is mild enough to use daily, if you like. When kept in a cool, dry place, this scrub stays fresh for up to 2 months.

1 cup dried peppermint leaves, packed

¾ cup baking soda

1. In a food processer or blender, combine the peppermint leaves and the baking soda. Process until a fine powder results.
2. Transfer the blend to a clean container with a tight-fitting lid.
3. Wet your face and use 1 teaspoon of the scrub to massage your skin, using light pressure and making tight circles. Rinse after you have covered all areas. Repeat once or twice per day.

# Poison Ivy

*"Leaflets three, let them be!" Try as you might to follow this wise old adage, a run-in with poison ivy can leave you with a painful, itchy rash that can take a long time to heal. Herbs can help you feel more comfortable while speeding the healing process.*

## Herbal Spray with Calendula, Chickweed, Chamomile, and Comfrey

Makes about 1 cup

This quick spray is easy to make with preformulated ingredients. Calendula, chickweed, chamomile, and comfrey combine with witch hazel to ease the itching, inflammation, and swelling that accompany poison ivy, while helping your skin heal faster. This spray will stay fresh for up to a year when stored in the refrigerator.

¼ cup witch hazel

2 tablespoons calendula oil

2 tablespoons chamomile tincture

2 tablespoons chickweed tincture

2 tablespoons comfrey tincture

1. In a dark-colored glass bottle with a spray top, combine all the ingredients. Shake gently to blend completely.
2. Apply 1 or 2 spritzes to each area where poison ivy is a concern. Repeat three or four times per day, and allow the spray to dry before dressing.

**Precautions** Omit the chamomile if you are allergic to plants in the ragweed family.

# Licorice Root Powder

Makes about 1 cup

Licorice contains two strong anti-inflammatory agents that act like the corticosteroids found in hydrocortisone. Called glycyrrhetic acid and glycyrrhizin, they help stop itching and inflammation quickly. The oatmeal helps soothe the itch, too, while allowing the licorice root to cling to your skin. Use this remedy within 2 weeks.

4 ounces dried licorice root

4 ounces organic rolled oats

1. In a food processor, combine the licorice root and rolled oats. Pulse to chop the licorice root into smaller pieces, then set the processor to high speed until the licorice root and rolled oats form a fine powder.
2. Transfer the finished powder to a clean, dry container with a tight-fitting lid and store in a cool, dry place.
3. With a cosmetic brush, apply a generous dusting of powder to the rash. Wear comfortable, breathable clothing over the powder. Reapply three to four times per day, with a final application just before bed.

**Precautions** Do not use licorice if you have high blood pressure, diabetes, kidney problems, or heart disease.

# Premenstrual Syndrome (PMS)

*Irritability, mood swings, bloating, and headaches are among the most common PMS symptoms. While the mental and physical discomfort that arises before the onset of a woman's monthly period are normal, it can be a struggle. These remedies help relieve the symptoms.*

## Dandelion-Ginger Tea

Makes 1 cup

Dandelion addresses the bloating that often accompanies PMS, while ginger eases cramps and gives your mood a little boost. If you like the taste of this tea and want to drink it frequently, you can easily make a large batch. Keep it in a pitcher in the refrigerator, and it will stay fresh for up to a week.

1 cup boiling water

1 teaspoon chopped dandelion root

1 teaspoon chopped gingerroot

1. Pour the boiling water into a large mug. Add the roots, cover the mug, and allow the tea to steep for 10 minutes.
2. Relax and drink the tea slowly while inhaling the steam. Repeat up to four times per day.

**Precautions** Do not use ginger if you take prescription blood thinners, have gallbladder disease, or have a bleeding disorder.

# Black Cohosh Syrup

Makes about 2 cups

Black cohosh helps balance hormonal activity, making it a little easier for you to deal with PMS symptoms. This slightly bitter syrup is a convenient alternative to tea, and it lasts for up to 6 months when stored in the refrigerator.

2 ounces black cohosh

2 cups water

1 cup honey

1. In a saucepan, combine the black cohosh and water. Bring the liquid to a simmer over low heat, cover partially with a lid, and reduce the liquid by half.
2. Transfer the contents of the saucepan to a glass measuring cup, then pour the mixture through a dampened piece of cheesecloth back into the saucepan, wringing the cheesecloth until no more liquid comes out.
3. Add the honey and warm the mixture over low heat, stirring constantly and stopping when the temperature reaches 105°F to 110°F.
4. Pour the syrup into a sterilized jar or bottle and store it in the refrigerator.
5. Take 1 tablespoon orally three times per day when PMS symptoms are a problem.

# Prostatitis

*With an inflamed prostate gland comes the need to urinate frequently—often with severe discomfort and sometimes with urethral discharge as well as low back pain. Because prostatitis symptoms are similar to those of other, more serious illnesses, be sure to obtain a professional diagnosis before moving forward with herbal treatments. Your doctor may also recommend antibiotics if an infection is present.*

## Hops Tea

Makes 1 cup

Hops contains xanthohumol, a substance that has been proven to possess anti-carcinogenic properties, particularly with regard to the prostate. It can also help alleviate benign prostate hyperplasia symptoms. Since sugar can aggravate prostatitis, sweeten this tea with stevia if you find the taste disagreeable. If tea is inconvenient, find a high-quality hops supplement and take it as recommended.

1 cup boiling water

1 teaspoon crumbled hops

1. Pour the boiling water into a large mug. Add the hops, cover the mug, and allow the tea to steep for 10 minutes.
2. Relax and drink the tea slowly while inhaling the steam. Hops can help you go to sleep faster at night, so consider enjoying this treatment at bedtime.

**Precautions** Do not give hops to prepubescent children of either gender.

# Turmeric-Saw Palmetto Tincture

Makes about 2 cups

Turmeric and saw palmetto reduce the pain and inflammation that accompany prostatitis. Taken daily, this tincture can help improve your quality of life. If you don't want to take a tincture, you can take high-quality supplements; they're easy to find at health food stores and drugstores. This tincture stays fresh for up to 6 years when kept in a cool, dark place.

4 ounces turmeric root, finely chopped

4 ounces saw palmetto, finely chopped

2 cups unflavored 80-proof vodka

1. In a sterilized pint jar, combine the herbs. Add the vodka, filling the jar to the very top and covering the herbs completely.
2. Cap the jar tightly and shake it up. Store it in a cool, dark cabinet and shake it several times per week for 6 to 8 weeks. If any of the alcohol evaporates, add more vodka so that the jar is again full to the top.
3. Dampen a piece of cheesecloth and drape it over the mouth of a funnel. Pour the tincture through the funnel into another sterilized pint jar. Squeeze the liquid from the herbs, wringing the cheesecloth until no more liquid comes out. Discard the spent herbs and transfer the finished tincture to dark-colored glass bottles.
4. Take 1 teaspoon orally twice per day. If the taste is too strong for you, you can mix it into a glass of water or juice and drink it.

**Precautions** Do not use turmeric if you have hypoglycemia.

# Psoriasis

*Psoriasis is a chronic skin condition with ups and downs that often accompany high and low stress levels. While stress management can help you keep breakouts to a minimum, soothing herbal treatments reduce the itching, pain, redness, and thick flaky patches of skin.*

## Licorice Root Spray

Makes 1 cup

With a pair of strong anti-inflammatory agents that act like the corticosteroids found in pharmaceuticals, licorice helps put a stop to itching and inflammation. The witch hazel in this recipe helps ease the itch, too.

¾ cup witch hazel

¼ cup licorice root tincture

1. In a dark-colored glass bottle with a spray top, combine the ingredients. Shake gently to blend completely.
2. Apply 1 or 2 spritzes to each area where psoriasis is a concern. Repeat three or four times per day whenever you are having a flare-up.

**Precautions** Do not use licorice if you have high blood pressure, diabetes, kidney problems, or heart disease.

# Goldenseal, Chamomile, and Comfrey Salve

Makes about 1 cup

Goldenseal, chamomile, and comfrey soothe pain and itching while offering anti-inflammatory benefits. Chamomile has a mild corticosteroid-like effect that is particularly effective against itching. This salve will stay fresh for up to a year when kept in a cool, dry place.

1 ounce dried goldenseal root, chopped

1 ounce dried chamomile

1 ounce dried comfrey

1 cup coconut oil

1 ounce beeswax

1. In a slow cooker, combine the herbs and coconut oil. Select the lowest heat setting, cover the slow cooker, and allow the herbs to steep in the oil for 3 to 5 hours. Turn off the heat and allow the infused oil to cool.

2. Bring an inch or so of water to a simmer in the base of a double boiler. Reduce the heat to low.

3. Drape a cheesecloth over the upper part of the double boiler. Pour in the infused oil, then wring and twist the cheesecloth until no more oil comes out. Discard the cheesecloth and spent herbs.

4. Add the beeswax to the infused oil and place the double boiler on the base. Gently warm over low heat. When the beeswax melts completely, remove the pan from the heat. Quickly pour the salve into clean, dry jars or tins and allow it to cool completely before capping.

5. With a cotton cosmetic pad or your fingertips, apply a dime-size amount to each area where psoriasis is a concern, using a little more or less as needed. Repeat three or four times per day, with a final application at bedtime.

**Precautions** Do not use goldenseal if you are pregnant or breastfeeding, or have high blood pressure. Avoid chamomile if you are allergic to plants in the ragweed family.

# Rheumatoid Arthritis

*Rheumatoid arthritis is different from osteoarthritis in that it is an immune inflammatory response rather than a condition caused by wear and tear. It affects joint linings and causes painful swelling, and you may also experience weakness or an overall sense of fatigue.*

## Blue Vervain-Comfrey Liniment

**Makes ½ cup**

Blue vervain and comfrey provide reliable pain relief and promote better circulation. If you have rosemary essential oil on hand, you can add it to the blend to increase its potency. This convenient liniment stays fresh for up to 7 years when kept in a cool, dry place.

⅓ cup unflavored 80-proof vodka

1 tablespoon blue vervain tincture

1 tablespoon comfrey tincture

20 drops rosemary essential oil (optional)

1. In a dark-colored glass bottle, combine the ingredients by shaking gently.
2. With a cotton cosmetic pad, apply 5 to 10 drops to the affected area. Use a little more or less as needed. Repeat as often as needed for pain relief.

**Precautions** Do not use blue vervain if you are pregnant. Do not use rosemary if you have epilepsy.

# Ginger-Licorice Salve

**Makes about 1 cup**

Ginger and licorice soothe the pain of rheumatoid arthritis while also promoting better circulation. This salve will stay fresh for up to a year when stored in a cool, dark place.

1 ounce dried gingerroot, chopped

1 ounce dried licorice root, chopped

1 cup light olive oil

1 ounce beeswax

1. In a slow cooker, combine the ginger, licorice, and olive oil. Select the lowest heat setting, cover the slow cooker, and allow the herbs to steep in the oil for 3 to 5 hours. Turn off the heat and allow the infused oil to cool.

2. Bring an inch or so of water to a simmer in the base of a double boiler. Reduce the heat to low.

3. Drape a piece of cheesecloth over the upper part of the double boiler. Pour in the infused oil, then wring and twist the cheesecloth until no more oil comes out. Discard the cheesecloth and spent herbs.

4. Add the beeswax to the infused oil and place the double boiler on the base. Gently warm over low heat. When the beeswax melts completely, remove the pan from the heat. Quickly pour the salve into clean, dry jars or tins and allow it to cool completely before capping.

5. With your fingertips, apply a dime-size amount of salve to affected areas, gently massaging. Use a little more or less as needed, and repeat as often as you like to keep discomfort in check.

**Precautions** Do not use ginger if you take prescription blood thinners, have gallbladder disease, or have a bleeding disorder. Do not use licorice if you have high blood pressure, diabetes, kidney problems, or heart disease.

# Ringworm

*Despite its name, ringworm isn't caused by a parasite. Instead, it's a fungal infection that shows up in the form of red, circular patches with raised, blister-like edges. Highly contagious and extremely itchy, ringworm spreads quickly from person to person; even your pets can get it. Be scrupulous with hygiene if you get it, and keep the area clean and dry while antifungal herbs do their work.*

## Fresh Garlic Compress

Makes 1 compress

Garlic is a strong antifungal agent that stops ringworm quickly. If you notice that a certain area is beginning to itch and tingle but no ringworm rash has appeared, you may be able to stop the rash from forming by applying fresh garlic to that spot.

1 cup steaming-hot water (not boiling)

1 garlic clove, cut in half

1. Soak a soft cloth in the hot water.
2. Press or purée half of the garlic clove and apply the paste to the area. Cover it with the cloth and apply a bandage to hold the treatment in place. Alternatively, if you're short on time, position half of the garlic clove over the ringworm rash, cut-side down. Cover it with the cloth and then wrap the area with a bandage.
3. Leave the compress in place for 10 to 15 minutes, then discard the garlic. Use a new piece of garlic for each area of ringworm.
4. Repeat the treatment two or three times per day until the ringworm is gone.

**Precautions** Garlic can cause skin irritation in sensitive individuals. Discontinue use if this occurs.

# Goldenseal Balm

**Makes ½ cup**

Goldenseal is a potent antifungal agent that also offers anti-inflammatory benefits to help stop the itching associated with ringworm. The coconut oil in this recipe also offers antifungal properties, and it will help your skin heal faster. If you have tea tree essential oil on hand, you can add it to this recipe to make the balm even stronger.

2 ounces dried goldenseal root

¼ cup coconut oil

½ ounce beeswax

20 drops tea tree essential oil (optional)

1. In a slow cooker, combine the goldenseal and coconut oil. Select the lowest heat setting, cover the slow cooker, and allow the herbs to steep in the oil for 3 to 5 hours. Turn off the heat and allow the infused oil to cool.

2. Bring an inch or so of water to a simmer in the base of a double boiler. Reduce the heat to low.

3. Drape a piece of cheesecloth over the upper half of the double boiler. Pour in the infused oil, then wring the cheesecloth until no more oil comes out. Discard the spent herbs.

4. Add the beeswax to the infused oil and place the double boiler on the base. Gently warm over low heat. When the beeswax melts completely, remove the pan from the heat. Add the tea tree essential oil (if using). Quickly pour the salve into clean, dry jars or tins and allow it to cool completely before capping.

5. With a cotton cosmetic pad or gauze pad, apply a pea-size amount of the balm to each area where ringworm is a concern. Repeat three or four times per day, with a final application at bedtime. Continue the treatment until the ringworm is gone.

**Precautions** Do not use goldenseal if you are pregnant or breastfeeding, or have high blood pressure.

# Rosacea

*A common, chronic skin disorder that usually begins as a tendency to flush or blush more often than average, rosacea often causes broken facial capillaries and small, pus-filled bumps. Usually affecting the nose and cheeks, rosacea sometimes spreads farther, affecting the forehead, chin, chest, and back.*

## Chamomile-Aloe Scrub

Makes 1 treatment

Chamomile and aloe ease inflammation, while oatmeal offers soothing properties of its own. If you like this treatment and want to use it a few times per week, you can mix a larger batch of chamomile and oat flour in equal proportions and then measure out 1 teaspoon of the blend to use with 1 teaspoon of aloe gel.

1 teaspoon aloe vera gel

½ teaspoon ground chamomile

½ teaspoon oat flour

1. In the palm of your hand, combine all the ingredients and apply the entire amount to your freshly washed face using gentle circular motions. Massage lightly, focusing on areas where rosacea is present.
2. Rinse your face with cool water and pat it dry. Repeat three or four times per week.

**Precautions** Do not use chamomile if you are allergic to plants in the ragweed family.

# Licorice-Feverfew Mask

**Makes ½ cup**

Licorice and feverfew offer strong anti-inflammatory benefits, as does the honey that helps these herbs cling to your skin. This sticky mask offers deep hydration, and is most conveniently applied in the shower. When kept in a cool, dark place, it will remain fresh for up to a year.

⅓ cup raw honey

1 tablespoon feverfew tincture

1 tablespoon licorice root tincture

1. Bring an inch or so of water to a simmer in the base of a double boiler. Reduce the heat to low.
2. In a glass measuring cup, combine all the ingredients. Place the measuring cup in the upper part of the double boiler and allow it to gently warm over low heat so that the honey's consistency becomes thinner.
3. With a small whisk, stir the blend to combine it completely. Quickly transfer it to a dark-colored glass bottle or jar.
4. Apply 1 to 2 teaspoons of the blend to your moistened face and leave it in place for 5 to 10 minutes, then rinse with cool water. Repeat three to four times per week.

**Precautions** Do not use feverfew if you are allergic to plants in the ragweed family. Do not use licorice if you have high blood pressure, diabetes, kidney problems, or heart disease.

# Shingles

*Indicated by a painful rash that usually affects the trunk area, shingles is caused when the same virus responsible for chicken pox reactivates. The pain can persist even after the blisters fade, leading to even more frustration.*

## Licorice Salve

Makes 1 cup

Licorice is an antiviral herb, plus it can aid in recovery from chronic stress and anxiety. Coconut oil is antiviral, too, and it helps damaged skin heal quickly. The salve will remain fresh for up to a year when kept in a cool, dark place.

4 ounces dried licorice root, chopped

1 cup coconut oil

1. In a slow cooker, combine the licorice root and coconut oil. Select the lowest heat setting, cover the slow cooker, and allow the herbs to steep in the oil for 3 to 5 hours. Turn off the heat. Cool.
2. Drape a piece of cheesecloth over a bowl. Pour in the infused oil, then wring the cheesecloth until no more oil comes out. Discard the spent herbs. Quickly pour the salve into clean, dry jars or tins and allow it to cool before capping.
3. With a cotton cosmetic pad, apply a dime-size amount to the shingles. Use a little more or less as needed, and repeat three or four times per day while symptoms are present.

**Precautions** Do not use licorice if you have high blood pressure, diabetes, or kidney or heart disease.

# Goldenseal-Comfrey Spray

Makes 1 cup

Soothing goldenseal and comfrey help skin heal faster, plus they offer antiviral benefits that may help shorten the duration of your shingles outbreak. Witch hazel provides cooling comfort. This spray will stay fresh for up to a year when kept refrigerated.

1 ounce dried comfrey

1 ounce dried goldenseal root

¼ cup fractionated coconut oil

¾ cup witch hazel

1. In a slow cooker, combine the comfrey, goldenseal, and fractionated coconut oil. Select the lowest heat setting, cover the slow cooker, and allow the herbs to steep in the oil for 3 to 5 hours. Turn off the heat and allow the infused oil to cool.
2. Drape a piece of cheesecloth over a bowl. Pour in the infused oil, then wring and twist the cheesecloth until no more oil comes out. Discard the cheesecloth and spent herbs.
3. In a dark-colored glass bottle with a spray top, combine the infused coconut oil with the witch hazel. Shake gently to blend completely.
4. Apply 1 or 2 spritzes to each area where shingles is a concern. Repeat as often as you like throughout each day of an outbreak.

**Precautions** Omit the goldenseal if you are pregnant or breastfeeding, or have high blood pressure.

# Sinus Infection

*The pain, postnasal drip, and pressure accompanying a sinus infection can make life seem unbearable. Often secondary to another condition such as allergies, this ailment often calls for a course of antibiotics. Herbs can help soothe your symptoms while the prescription does its job, especially if you start using the herbs at the first sign of symptoms.*

## Horseradish Shot

Makes 1 treatment

Horseradish is pungent, but it clears blocked sinuses quickly, and its antibiotic properties support your immune system. If you don't mind a moment of discomfort on the palate, you'll like what this treatment does for you.

1 teaspoon fresh or prepared horseradish
  or wasabi

2 tablespoons water

1. In a small glass, combine the horseradish and the water.
2. Drink the blend quickly. Repeat up to three times per day while fighting a sinus infection or treating a cold.

**Precautions** Do not use horseradish if you have low thyroid function or take thyroxine.

# Peppermint-Echinacea Tea

Makes 1 cup

This soothing tea supports your immune system while warming and soothing sore sinuses. Breathing the fragrant steam will help almost as much as drinking the tea will.

1 cup boiling water

1 teaspoon dried peppermint

1 teaspoon chopped dried echinacea root

1. Pour the boiling water into a large mug. Add the dried herbs, cover the mug, and allow the tea to steep for 10 minutes.
2. Relax and drink the tea slowly while inhaling the steam. Repeat up to four times per day.

**Precautions** Do not use echinacea if you are allergic to ragweed or if you have an autoimmune disorder.

# Skin Tag

*Skin tags, benign growths that start out as tiny bumps, can grow to uncomfortable proportions if left unchecked. If you experience repeated skin tags in a particular area, check for friction, as this is believed to be their primary cause. Treatment with herbal remedies can help you get rid of small skin tags, but larger ones often require medical intervention.*

## Ginger Poultice

Makes about ¼ cup

Fresh ginger is an excellent treatment for skin tags. Its healing properties shrink the tag, leaving you with smooth, clear skin. You can easily double this recipe to last all week.

4 ounces fresh gingerroot

1. In a food processer or blender, process the ginger until a fine paste forms.
2. Clean and dry the skin tag. Use your fingertip or a cotton swab to apply the ginger to the skin tag, ensuring that you cover the entire thing. Cover the skin tag with a disposable bandage or a piece of tape.
3. Repeat twice per day until the skin tag falls off. The amount of time will vary depending on the strength of the ginger poultice and the size of your skin tag.

**Precautions** If you notice irritation anywhere other than the skin tag, discontinue use.

# Fresh Dandelion Sap

Makes 1 treatment

The sap from a freshly picked dandelion flower's stem dries and irritates small skin tags, making them shrivel. Be absolutely sure that the dandelions you use for this treatment have not been treated with pesticides or herbicides.

1 dandelion flower with stem

Light olive oil or coconut oil

1. Using your thumb and pointer finger, use one smooth motion to squeeze (as you would with a tube of toothpaste) the sap from a cut dandelion stem into a small dish.
2. With a cotton swab or your fingertip, apply a thin layer of olive oil or coconut oil to the skin beneath the skin tag. This acts as a barrier, preventing the dandelion sap from contacting healthy skin.
3. Use your cotton swab or fingertip to apply the sap to the skin tag, ensuring that you cover the entire thing. Cover the skin tag with a disposable bandage or a piece of tape.
4. Repeat once or twice per day until the skin tag falls off. The amount of time will vary depending on the strength of the sap and the size of your skin tag.

# Sore Muscles

*Usually caused by overwork or even by sitting in the same position for too long, sore muscles take time to heal. Herbs can ease the pain and help you relax, while taking it easy for a day or two will promote faster healing.*

## Ginger-Fennel Massage Oil

**Makes 1 cup**

Fennel and ginger offer a pleasant, warming effect that soothes and relaxes tight, sore muscles. This treatment will stay fresh for up to 6 months when kept in a cool, dark place.

1 tablespoon crushed fennel seeds

2 ounces dried gingerroot, chopped

1 cup light olive oil

1. In a slow cooker, combine the fennel, ginger, and olive oil. Select the lowest heat setting, cover the slow cooker, and allow the herbs to steep in the oil for 3 to 5 hours. Turn off the heat and allow the infused oil to cool.
2. Drape a piece of cheesecloth over a bowl. Pour in the infused oil, then wring and twist the cheesecloth until no more oil comes out. Discard the cheesecloth and spent herbs.
3. Transfer the oil to a dark-colored bottle with a tight-fitting lid.
4. With your fingertips, apply 1 teaspoon to affected areas, using a little more or less oil as needed. Massage using moderate pressure. Repeat as often as needed to provide drug-free pain relief.

**Precautions** Do not use ginger if you take prescription blood thinners, have gallbladder disease, or have a bleeding disorder.

# Peppermint-St. John's Wort Salve

Makes about 1 cup

Peppermint and St. John's wort provide deep pain relief while helping muscles relax. Be careful with this remedy when it is finished, since the red color of the St. John's wort can stain clothing. When stored in a cool, dark place, this salve stays fresh for up to a year.

1 cup light olive oil

2 ounces St. John's wort

1 ounce dried peppermint

1 ounce beeswax

1. In a slow cooker, combine the olive oil, St. John's wort, and peppermint. Select the lowest heat setting, cover the slow cooker, and allow the herbs to steep in the oil for 3 to 5 hours. Turn off the heat and allow the infused oil to cool.
2. Bring an inch or so of water to a simmer in the base of a double boiler. Reduce the heat to low.
3. Drape a piece of cheesecloth over the upper part of the double boiler. Pour in the infused oil, then wring and twist the cheesecloth until no more oil comes out. Discard the cheesecloth and spent herbs.
4. Add the beeswax to the infused oil and place the double boiler on the base. Gently warm over low heat. When the beeswax melts completely, remove the blend from the heat. Quickly pour the salve into clean, dry jars or tins and allow it to cool completely before capping.
5. With your fingertips, apply a dime-size amount of the salve to the affected area, using a little more or less as needed. Repeat as often as needed for pain relief.

**Precautions** Do not use St. John's wort if you take a monoamine oxidase inhibitor (MAOI) or selective serotonin reuptake inhibitor (SSRI).

# Sore Throat

*Whether your sore throat is associated with a virus, allergies, dry air, or airborne irritants, the pain can make you feel miserable. Although herbal remedies can be effective, you may need antibiotics if a bacterial infection is present. If you suspect that strep throat is to blame, see your doctor immediately.*

## Peppermint Tea with Comfrey and Sage

### Makes 1 cup

Peppermint, comfrey, and sage ease the pain of a sore throat, and the warmth of the tea provides additional relief from inflammation. Add honey and lemon to taste if you find that the flavor of this tea is too strong for you.

1 cup boiling water

1 teaspoon dried peppermint

1 teaspoon dried comfrey

1 teaspoon dried sage

1. Pour the boiling water into a large mug. Add the dried herbs, cover the mug, and allow the tea to steep for 10 minutes.
2. Inhale deeply while relaxing and sipping the tea. Repeat up to four times per day as needed.

# Agrimony-Licorice Gargle

Makes 1 cup

Agrimony, licorice, and honey provide soothing pain relief. If you like, you can drink this gargle as a tea. Or if you think that you'd like a cool sensation, refrigerate it before use.

1 cup boiling water

1 tablespoon agrimony

1 teaspoon chopped licorice root

1 teaspoon honey

1. Pour the boiling water into a large mug. Add the herbs and honey, cover the mug, and allow the blend to steep for 10 minutes.
2. Let the liquid cool to room temperature. Gargle with 1 tablespoon at a time, repeating as often as needed to bring relief from throat pain.

**Precautions** Do not use licorice if you have high blood pressure, diabetes, kidney problems, or heart disease.

# Sprain

*Minor sprains respond best to compression, elevation, ice, and rest. But herbs can help promote circulation while easing the pain. If you have a severe sprain with bruising and swelling, be sure to see your doctor as soon as possible—what you think is just a bad sprain could actually be far worse.*

## Arnica Gel

Makes ½ cup

Arnica offers fast, reliable pain relief and does a remarkable job of reducing bruising and swelling around sprains. This simple gel is easy to make and lasts for up to a year when stored in the refrigerator.

⅓ cup aloe vera gel

2 tablespoons arnica tincture

1. In a small bowl, combine the aloe vera gel and the arnica tincture. Use a fork or whisk to blend it completely. Transfer the gel to a clean container with a tight-fitting lid.
2. With your fingers or a cotton cosmetic pad, apply a dime-size amount of the gel to your sprain. Use a little more or less gel as needed, and allow it to penetrate the site completely before bandaging or dressing. Repeat two or three times per day while recovering.

**Precautions** Do not use arnica on open or bleeding wounds. Skin irritation can occur with long-term use; discontinue if a rash develops.

# Comfrey-Ginger Balm and Compress

## Makes about 1 cup

Comfrey and ginger soothe pain quickly while promoting good circulation at the injured site. Topping this balm with a cold compress will help reduce swelling. The balm is a good one for a variety of aches and pains, and will remain fresh for up to a year when stored in a cool, dark place.

1 ounce dried comfrey

1 ounce dried gingerroot, chopped

1 cup light olive oil

1 ounce beeswax

1. In a slow cooker, combine the comfrey, ginger, and olive oil. Select the lowest heat setting, cover the slow cooker, and allow the herbs to steep in the oil for 3 to 5 hours. Turn off the heat and allow the infused oil to cool.

2. Bring an inch of water to a simmer in the base of a double boiler. Reduce the heat to low.

3. Drape a cheesecloth over the upper part of the double boiler. Pour in the infused oil, then wring the cheesecloth until no more oil comes out. Discard the spent herbs.

4. Add the beeswax to the infused oil and place the double boiler on the base. Gently warm over low heat. When the beeswax melts, remove the pan from the heat. Quickly pour the salve into clean, dry jars or tins and allow it to cool completely before capping.

5. With your fingertips, apply a dime-size amount of balm to the injured area, using a little more or less as needed. Allow the balm to melt into your skin for a minute or two, then top it with an ice pack wrapped in a tea towel. Leave the cold compress in place for 10 to 15 minutes, removing it if your skin starts to feel numb. Repeat every 1 to 2 hours while recovering.

**Precautions**  Do not use ginger if you take prescription blood thinners, have gallbladder disease, or have a bleeding disorder.

# Stiff Joints

*Freezing temperatures, old injuries, and osteoarthritis are a few things that lead to stiff, achy joints. While herbs can make you more comfortable, they will not cure you permanently. Be sure to talk with your doctor if your pain is long lasting or severe.*

## Peppermint-Comfrey Massage Oil

**Makes 1 cup**

Peppermint and comfrey deliver penetrating pain relief and help improve circulation. This remedy takes a little time to make, but it stays fresh for up to a year when stored in a cool, dark place.

1 ounce dried peppermint

1 ounce dried comfrey

1 cup jojoba oil

1. In a slow cooker, combine the peppermint, comfrey, and jojoba oil. Select the lowest heat setting, cover the slow cooker, and allow the herbs to steep in the oil for 3 to 5 hours. Turn off the heat and allow the infused oil to cool.
2. Drape a piece of cheesecloth over a bowl. Pour in the infused oil, then wring and twist the cheesecloth until no more oil comes out. Discard the cheesecloth and spent herbs.
3. Transfer the massage oil to a bottle with a tight-fitting lid.
4. With a cotton cosmetic pad or your fingertips, apply ½ teaspoon to the affected area, using a little more or less as needed. Using gentle pressure, massage using circular motions. Repeat two or three times per day to relieve stiff, sore joints and muscles.

# Horseradish Salve

Makes about 1 cup

Beyond its usefulness as a condiment and natural decongestant, horseradish offers topical pain relief while warming joints and muscles. It also increases circulation, helping to ease inflammation and prolong relief. This salve will remain fresh for up to a year when kept in a cool, dark place.

2 ounces horseradish root, grated

1 cup light olive oil

1 ounce beeswax

1. In a slow cooker, combine the horse-radish and olive oil. Select the lowest heat setting, cover the slow cooker, and allow the herbs to steep in the oil for 6 to 12 hours. Turn off the heat and allow the infused oil to cool.

2. Bring an inch or so of water to a simmer in the base of a double boiler. Reduce the heat to low.

3. Drape a piece of cheesecloth over the upper part of the double boiler. Pour in the infused oil, then wring and twist the cheesecloth until no more oil comes out. Discard the cheesecloth and spent herbs.

4. Add the beeswax to the infused oil and place the double boiler on the base. Gently warm over low heat. When the beeswax melts completely, remove the pan from the heat. Quickly pour the salve into clean, dry jars or tins and allow it to cool completely before capping.

5. With a cotton cosmetic pad or your fin-gertips, apply a dime-size amount of salve to the affected area. Massage it in gently. Repeat one or two times per day as needed.

**Precautions** Do not use if you have low thyroid function or take thyroxine. Overuse may blister skin; discontinue if this occurs.

# Sunburn

*While prevention is best, sunburn happens even to people who are cautious. If you're having trouble sleeping because of the discomfort, consider taking an herbal sedative in addition to using the topical remedies outlined here. Be sure to seek medical attention if your sunburn is severe, with blisters, serious pain, or signs of infection.*

## Comfrey Spray

Makes about 1 cup

This quick comfrey spray soothes the sting of a sunburn quickly, thanks to the anti-inflammatory benefits of the comfrey tincture and the witch hazel. When kept refrigerated, it will stay fresh for up to a year.

1 cup witch hazel

2 tablespoons comfrey tincture

1. In a dark-colored glass bottle with a spray top, combine the witch hazel and comfrey tincture. Shake gently to blend completely.
2. Apply 1 or 2 spritzes to each sunburned area, using more or less as needed. Allow the spray to dry before dressing, and wear soft, breathable clothing. Repeat three or four times per day until your sunburn heals.

# Hyssop-Infused Aloe Vera Gel

Makes about ½ cup

Hyssop and aloe vera gel can comfort your sunburn while promoting faster healing. If you don't feel like making a hyssop decoction and you have hyssop tincture on hand, you can use 1 tablespoon of it in place of the infusion. This gel stays fresh for up to 2 weeks in the refrigerator.

2 tablespoons dried hyssop

½ cup water

¼ cup aloe vera gel

1. In a saucepan, combine the hyssop and water. Bring the mixture to a boil over high heat, then reduce the heat to low. Simmer the mixture until it reduces by half, then remove it from the heat and allow it to cool completely.

2. Dampen a piece of cheesecloth and drape it over the mouth of a funnel. Pour the mixture through the funnel into a glass bowl. Squeeze the liquid from the herbs, wringing the cheesecloth until no more liquid comes out.

3. Add the aloe vera gel to the liquid and use a whisk to blend. Transfer the finished gel to a sterilized glass jar. Cap the jar tightly and store it in the refrigerator.

4. With a cotton cosmetic pad or your fingertips, apply a thin layer to all affected areas three or four times per day.

**Precautions** Do not use hyssop if you are pregnant or have epilepsy.

# Tendinitis

*Repetitive actions and impacts can lead to irritation or inflammation in the bands of tissue that connect your muscles to your bones. Common locations include the elbow, shoulder, thumb, knee, and Achilles tendon. Herbs help soothe the discomfort, and it's important to rest so the body can heal. Physical therapy might be needed in severe cases.*

## Ginger-Turmeric Tea

Makes 1 cup

Ginger and turmeric decrease inflammation, ease pain, and promote better circulation while helping you relax so you can recover a bit faster. Add a little honey and lemon to flavor this tea if you like.

1 cup boiling water

1 tablespoon chopped fresh gingerroot

1 teaspoon ground turmeric

1. Pour the boiling water into a large mug. Add the ginger and turmeric, cover the mug, and allow the tea to steep for 10 minutes.
2. Relax and drink the tea slowly. Repeat up to four times per day.

**Precautions** Do not use ginger if you take prescription blood thinners, or have a bleeding disorder or gallbladder disease. If you have hypoglycemia, you can use small amounts of turmeric as a culinary spice, but you should not take it in large amounts.

# Peppermint Salve

Makes about 1 cup

Peppermint penetrates deeply into tissue, providing a cooling sensation. Its analgesic properties make it an effective, all-natural pain reliever. If you have peppermint essential oil on hand, you can increase the potency of this salve significantly. Useful for a variety of muscle and joint complaints, peppermint salve will stay fresh for up to a year when kept in a cool, dark place.

2 ounces dried peppermint

1 cup light olive oil

1 ounce beeswax

20 to 30 drops peppermint essential oil (optional)

1. In a slow cooker, combine the peppermint and olive oil. Select the lowest heat setting, cover the slow cooker, and allow the herbs to steep in the oil for 3 to 5 hours. Turn off the heat and allow the infused oil to cool.
2. Bring an inch or so of water to a simmer in the base of a double boiler. Reduce the heat to low.
3. Drape a cheesecloth over the upper part of the double boiler. Pour in the infused oil, then wring and twist the cheesecloth until no more oil comes out. Discard the cheesecloth and spent herbs.
4. Add the beeswax to the infused oil and place the double boiler on the base. Gently warm over low heat. When the beeswax melts completely, remove the pan from the heat. Add the peppermint essential oil (if using). Quickly pour the salve into clean, dry jars or tins and allow it to cool completely before capping.
5. With your fingertips or a cotton cosmetic swab, apply a dime-size amount to the injured area. Use a little more or less as needed, and repeat every 2 to 3 hours while pain persists.

# Travel Sickness

*Call it motion sickness or seasickness; the symptoms are all the same. Severe nausea, dizziness, sweating, uneasiness, and even vomiting often respond well to herbal remedies. These treatments help you feel better so you can enjoy the journey with none of the side effects that accompany conventional remedies.*

## Chamomile Syrup

Makes 2 cups

Chamomile settles upset stomachs quickly, and is gentle enough for children to use. This remedy stays fresh for up to 6 months when refrigerated.

2 ounces dried chamomile

2 cups water

1 cup honey

1. In a saucepan, combine the chamomile and water. Bring the liquid to a simmer over low heat, cover partially with a lid, and reduce the liquid by half.
2. Transfer the mixture to a glass measuring cup, then pour it through a dampened piece of cheesecloth back into the saucepan, wringing the liquid from the cheesecloth.
3. Add the honey and warm the mixture over low heat, stirring constantly, until the temperature reaches 105°F to 110°F.
4. Pour the syrup into a sterilized jar or bottle and store it in the refrigerator.
5. Take 1 tablespoon orally three times per day, or more often as needed. Children under age 12 should take 1 teaspoon up to three times per day.

**Precautions** Avoid if you are allergic to plants in the ragweed family or taking prescription blood thinners.

# Candied Ginger

Makes about 1 pound

Candied ginger is easy to consume, and it's ideal for taking along while traveling. Ginger's ability to soothe motion sickness is legendary, making this treatment a reliable one that also happens to be delicious.

5 cups water

1 pound fresh gingerroot, peeled and cut into
⅛-inch-thick slices

1 pound raw cane sugar

1. Line a baking sheet with parchment. Spray a cooling rack with nonstick baking spray and place it on the baking sheet.
2. In a 4-quart saucepan, combine the water and ginger. Cover and cook over medium-high heat until the ginger is tender enough to be pierced with a fork, about 30 minutes.
3. Pour the cooking liquid into a pitcher to use for tea, if you like, or strain it into the sink, reserving ¼ cup.
4. Return the ginger and the reserved cooking water to the saucepan, add the sugar, and bring to a boil over medium-high heat, stirring frequently. Reduce the heat to medium and cook, stirring frequently, until the sugar begins to recrystallize, about 20 minutes.
5. Transfer the ginger to the rack and use tongs or a fork to separate the pieces. When completely cool, store the ginger in an airtight container for up to 2 weeks. If you like, you can wrap and freeze a portion for up to 6 months.
6. Enjoy pieces of ginger periodically while traveling. Eat as much as you like to keep motion sickness from settling in.

**Precautions** Do not use ginger if you take prescription blood thinners, have gallbladder disease, or have a bleeding disorder.

# Urinary Tract Infection (UTI)

*Painful urination, urgency, and frequent urination are key indicators of a urinary tract infection. Start herbal treatments as soon as you suspect that you might have a UTI, and you'll put a stop to symptoms faster. Be sure to stay well hydrated while caring for yourself. See your doctor if you develop a fever, or if your pain worsens or fails to subside.*

## Horseradish Tea

Makes 8 cups

Pungent but effective, horseradish is a strong antibacterial agent and diuretic that does double duty, killing bacteria and promoting urination to help the bladder flush faster. You will probably not like the way this tea tastes, but it can help you feel better.

½ cup grated fresh horseradish root

8 cups boiling water

1. In a saucepan, combine the horseradish and the boiling water. Cover the pot and allow the tea to steep for 10 minutes.
2. Cool the tea to at least room temperature. Pour an 8-ounce glass and drink it down quickly. Refrigerate the rest of the tea and continue drinking it throughout the day, consuming one glass every 2 hours or so. Drink lots of other liquids in between doses.

**Precautions** Do not use horseradish if you have low thyroid function or take thyroxine.

# Dandelion Tincture

**Makes about 2 cups**

Dandelion root is a diuretic that helps the bladder flush toxins faster. It also supports the liver, helping with detoxification in the event that you're taking antibiotics for your urinary tract infection. This tincture is a good digestive tonic, and you can use it as a gentle laxative, too. The tincture will stay fresh for up to 6 years when kept in a cool, dark place.

8 ounces dandelion root, finely chopped

2 cups unflavored 80-proof vodka

1. Put the dandelion root in a sterilized pint jar. Add the vodka, filling the jar to the very top and covering the herbs completely.

2. Cap the jar tightly and shake it up. Store it in a cool, dark cabinet and shake it several times per week for 6 to 8 weeks. If any of the alcohol evaporates, add more vodka so that the jar is again full to the top.

3. Dampen a piece of cheesecloth and drape it over the mouth of a funnel. Pour the tincture through the funnel into another sterilized pint jar. Squeeze the liquid from the herbs, wringing the cheesecloth until no more liquid comes out. Discard the spent herbs and transfer the finished tincture to dark-colored glass bottles.

4. Take 1/2 teaspoon orally three or four times per day while recovering. You can help your UTI even more by mixing the tincture into a tall glass of unsweetened cranberry juice.

# Warts

*Warts are caused by a virus that attacks the top layer of skin, causing rapid cell growth that leads to the formation of a lumpy, unsightly bump that might or might not itch. While herbal remedies can often eliminate small warts, large ones may need to be removed via conventional methods.*

## Fresh Basil Compress

Makes 1 treatment

Basil contains potent antiviral compounds that can help eliminate small warts. If you'd rather save your fresh basil for culinary use, you can use a drop or two of basil essential oil for this treatment instead.

1 teaspoon chopped fresh basil

1. Cover the wart with the chopped basil, then tape a square of linen or gauze over it. Leave the compress in place for 2 to 3 hours.
2. Remove the compress and rinse the area with cool water to remove the spent herb. Repeat the treatment up to three times per day until the wart is gone.

# Garlic Oil

### Makes ½ cup

Garlic is a very strong antiviral agent that can help get rid of warts quickly. This remedy takes longer to make than a fresh garlic compress does, but it saves you time and effort in the long run. If you also opt to cover the treated wart with raw honey, which also offers antiviral properties, your wart may disappear even faster. The infused oil will remain fresh for up to a year when kept in a cool, dark place.

4 ounces dried or freeze-dried garlic, chopped

¼ cup fractionated coconut oil

Raw honey (optional)

1. In a slow cooker, combine the garlic and coconut oil. Select the lowest heat setting, cover the slow cooker, and allow the herbs to steep in the oil for 3 to 5 hours. Turn off the heat and allow the infused oil to cool.
2. Drape a piece of cheesecloth over a bowl. Pour in the infused oil, then wring and twist the cheesecloth until no more oil comes out. Discard the cheesecloth and spent herbs.
3. Transfer the oil to a dark-colored bottle or jar.
4. With a cotton swab, apply 1 or 2 drops to the wart. Cover the wart with a drop of raw honey (if using), then cover the treated area with a disposable bandage.
5. Repeat the treatment two times per day, rinsing the treated area with cool water between applications, until the wart disappears.

**Precautions** Garlic can cause skin irritation in sensitive individuals. Discontinue use if irritation appears anywhere other than the wart.

# Weight Loss

*Obesity is a chronic condition that is far more than a simple cosmetic concern. It can compound other illnesses while making you feel uncomfortable in your own skin. It's true that a healthy, whole-foods diet and plenty of exercise are key to effective, lasting weight loss. It's also true that herbs can make the lifestyle change go more smoothly while promoting more efficient metabolism.*

## Dieter's Tea Blend with Chickweed, Dandelion, and Fennel

Makes 1 cup

Chickweed, dandelion, and fennel support weight loss by flushing toxins and helping you rid yourself of excess sodium that leads to bloating and water retention. Fennel also helps curb your appetite, making it a bit easier to resist cravings. This convenient tea blend stays fresh for up to 2 months when stored in a cool, dry place. You can add a bit of lemon juice to the hot tea if you like.

3 ounces dried chickweed

3 ounces dried dandelion root, chopped

3 ounces fennel seeds, crushed

1 cup boiling water

1. In a large container with a tight-fitting lid, combine the chickweed, dandelion root, and fennel.
2. Measure 2 teaspoons of the tea mixture into a large mug. Add the boiling water, cover the mug, and allow the herbs to steep for 10 minutes.
3. Drink the tea. Enjoy two or three cups per day while losing weight.

# Ginseng Tincture

Makes about 2 cups

Ginseng increases circulation, boosts your mood, and provides you with nutritional support while you are losing weight. It is a good source of vitamin $B_{12}$, which your body uses to manufacture red blood cells and transform your food to energy. This tincture is a good overall tonic, and will stay fresh for up to 6 years when kept in a cool, dry place.

8 ounces Panax ginseng or American ginseng, finely chopped

2 cups unflavored 80-proof vodka

1. Put the ginseng in a sterilized pint jar. Add the vodka, filling the jar to the very top and covering the herbs completely.
2. Cap the jar tightly and shake it up. Store it in a cool, dark cabinet and shake it several times per week for 6 to 8 weeks. If any of the alcohol evaporates, add more vodka so that the jar is again full to the top.
3. Dampen a piece of cheesecloth and drape it over the mouth of a funnel. Pour the tincture through the funnel into another sterilized pint jar. Squeeze the liquid from the herbs, wringing the cheesecloth until no more liquid comes out. Discard the spent herbs and transfer the finished tincture to dark-colored glass bottles.
4. Take ½ teaspoon orally each morning for 1 month, and then take 2 weeks off from the remedy. Repeat this cycle as many times as you like.

**Precautions** Do not use ginseng during pregnancy. Be sure to observe the 2-week rest period as recommended.

# Wrinkles

*A common sign of aging, wrinkles are far easier to prevent than they are to eliminate. Just as with cosmetics, herbs don't magically erase your crow's feet and light lines; they may, however, help you achieve smoother-looking skin naturally.*

## Calendula Toner

Makes ½ cup

This nourishing toner deeply moisturizes and refreshes your face. Calendula stimulates skin cell growth, helping to keep your complexion looking as smooth as possible. This toner stays fresh for up to a year when kept refrigerated.

⅓ cup witch hazel
2 tablespoons calendula oil

1. In a dark-colored glass bottle, combine the ingredients by shaking gently.
2. With a cotton cosmetic pad, apply 5 or 6 drops to your freshly washed face. Use a little more or less as needed.
3. Repeat twice per day. Consider doing one treatment as you get ready for the day and enjoying the second while you're preparing to go to bed.

# Aloe Gel Facial

Makes 1 treatment

Aloe vera gel nourishes skin and plumps up thirsty cells, reducing the appearance of fine lines and wrinkles. The coconut oil used in the second step of this treatment helps the skin shed dead, dull cells faster, for a smoother-looking complexion.

1 tablespoon aloe vera gel

1 teaspoon coconut oil

1.  Apply the aloe vera gel to your freshly washed face. Wait for it to absorb, then apply the coconut oil.
2.  Dampen a facial cloth with warm water. Relax and lay the cloth over your face. Leave it in place for 2 minutes, then remove it.
3.  Rinse your face with warm (not hot) water to remove any excess coconut oil. Repeat four times per week.

# Yeast Infection

*Also known as candidiasis, yeast infections happen when the Candida albicans organisms that normally populate the GI tract, skin, and vagina grow out of control. In some cases, a yeast infection is preceded by a course of prescription antibiotics that kills off the "good" bacteria that normally keep yeast in check.*

## Garlic Suppository

**Makes 6 treatments**

Garlic kills fungus quickly, and yogurt helps bring balance back to the vagina after a yeast infection. This treatment is messy and unpleasant, but it works very well. Be sure to protect your clothing by wearing panty liners during and after treatments.

6 garlic cloves, peeled

6 tablespoons plain yogurt with live,
    active cultures

1. In a mini food processer or blender, combine the garlic and yogurt and process until a smooth paste forms.
2. Transfer the paste to a clean, airtight container and refrigerate until you are ready to use it.
3. Use one-sixth of the remedy to coat an applicator-free tampon. Insert the tampon into your vagina and leave it in place for 1 hour. Remove and discard the tampon. Repeat the remedy twice a day for 3 days. Do not presoak the tampons, since this might make them swollen and difficult to put in place.

**Precautions** Garlic can cause severe skin irritation in sensitive individuals. Be absolutely sure that you are not sensitive to garlic before using this treatment. Discontinue if any irritation develops.

# Chamomile-Calendula Douche with Echinacea

### Makes 2 cups

Chamomile and calendula soothe the itch that comes with a yeast infection, while echinacea targets the yeast fungus. Unlike harsh chemical douche formulas, this one provides comfort without any potential for unwanted side effects.

4 cups water

1 tablespoon dried chamomile

1 tablespoon dried calendula

1 tablespoon chopped dried echinacea root

1. In a saucepan, combine the water, chamomile, calendula, and echinacea. Bring the mixture to a boil over high heat, then reduce the heat to low. Simmer the mixture until it reduces by half, then remove the pan from the heat. Allow it to cool completely. Refrigerate the blend until you are ready to use it.

2. While showering, use a douche to apply 1 cup of the blend to the vagina. Repeat the treatment once a day for 2 days.

**Precautions** Do not use if you are allergic to plants in the ragweed family; avoid if you are taking prescription blood thinners.

CHAPTER 4

# Herbs to Know

*Here you'll find 40 herbal medicine staples—from agrimony to witch hazel. This is by no means an exhaustive list of common herbs, as there are hundreds of safe, useful ones. However these are among the most accessible. All of them can be purchased in whole form, and many are easy to find in ready-to-use capsules, salves, tablets, teas, tinctures, and more.*

COST KEY

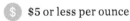

$ $5 or less per ounce

$ $ $5–$10 per ounce

$ $ $ $10 or more per ounce

# Agrimony

*Agrimonia eupatoria,*
*Agrimonia gryposepala*

*Until the late nineteenth century, agrimony was a common treatment for cough, diarrhea, skin conditions, and sore throat. This common, useful herb offers a slightly sweet scent that might remind you of apricots. It makes a pleasant addition to herbal teas, especially when you have a cold or the flu.*

**Parts Used:** Leaves and flowers

**Precautions:** Can aggravate constipation

**Identifying/Growing:** More commonly known as the cocklebur or sticklewort, agrimony is a member of the rose family. Instead of prickly thorns, its woody stem is covered in soft down. Toothy, dark green leaves adorn the branches, giving way to spikes of small, bright yellow flowers that leave prickly burrs behind when they fade. The plant reaches an average height of 2 feet, with some plants reaching 4 feet.

Though commonly found in fields and woodlands throughout Europe and North America, agrimony is easy to grow. It prefers full sun to partial shade, and requires moderate watering. The soil should be kept moist and well drained. Harvest the leaves anytime throughout the season, and snip the flowers when they begin to bloom.

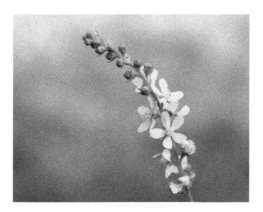

# Aloe

*Aloe vera, Aloe barbadensis,*
*Aloe ferox*

*Although aloe is a succulent that looks like a cactus, it is a member of the lily family. Its thick, spiky leaves are filled with a rich gel that's useful for treating burns, cuts, and scrapes. While fresh aloe is fantastic to have on hand, the bottled kind is also effective and convenient.*

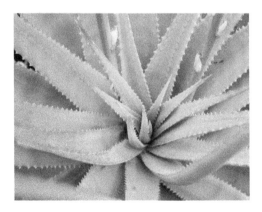

**Parts Used:** Gel and juice from inner leaves

**Precautions:** Aloe juice is a strong laxative. It should not be taken internally during pregnancy or while breastfeeding.

**Identifying/Growing:** There are over 250 aloe species worldwide. Most species are native to Africa, and feature intricate gray-green patterns on their leaves as well as tall, slender stems yielding yellow, tube-shaped flowers. You probably won't find this plant growing wild unless you live in a tropical climate, but you can easily grow it as a houseplant.

Plant your aloe in a wide pot filled with gravelly or sandy soil. Feed it with slow-release pellets or a 10-40-10 fertilizer, and water it regularly. Allow the soil to dry completely between waterings, particularly during the winter months when it has its dormancy phase. If you live in a cold area with warm summers, feel free to put your aloe outdoors when there is no chance of freezing weather.

# Angelica

*Angelica archangelica*

( $ )

*Angelica was traditionally used as a birthing herb for bringing on delayed labor. It is an excellent herb to aid with painful menstruation and cramps. Also, its ability to ease congestion and indigestion make it useful for treating the whole family.*

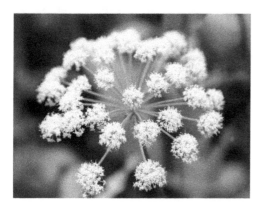

**Parts Used:** Root, leaves, stems, and fruit

**Precautions:** Angelica is a strong emmenagogue, meaning it increases blood flow in and to the pelvic area and uterus, even causing menstruation. It should not be used during pregnancy. It contains high levels of coumarin, a fragrant organic compound with blood-thinning properties, and can cause an adverse interaction with anticoagulant drugs.

**Identifying/Growing:** Angelica grows wild in fields and meadows throughout the world's temperate zones, particularly along streams and rivers. It prefers fairly shady areas, where you'll find it growing to a height of 3 to 6 feet. Clusters of small creamy yellow or greenish flowers emerge in late June to July and emit a lovely aroma.

You can grow angelica in a spot with partial shade to full sun. Moist, well-drained soil is ideal, as is proximity to a water feature. Place your plants at least 12 inches apart after germination, and harvest them when they are fully mature. Angelica is a biennial plant; planting it successively year after year will ensure that you get a harvest every year.

# Arnica

*Arnica Montana*

*Arnica is a beautiful alpine herb that offers such strong anti-inflammatory properties that it is well known even outside herbal medicine circles. While arnica creams and oils are convenient, the whole herb is also readily available online.*

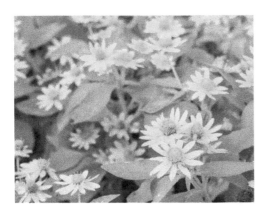

**Parts Used:** Flowers

**Precautions:** Do not use in open or bleeding wounds. Long-term use can cause skin irritation.

**Identifying/Growing:** Also known as mountain arnica, this aromatic herb can be found growing in alpine meadows. It features aromatic toothed leaves and bright yellow to orange blossoms with daisy-like florets on stalks that average 1 to 2 feet high.

Arnica prefers full sun but will tolerate a little shade. If you decide to grow this herb, you'll need patience since the seeds can take between 1 month and 2 years to germinate. You can either sow the seeds outside in late summer and hope for the best, or sow them in large pots indoors; they germinate at a temperature of about 55°F. Once the arnica begins to grow, it will flower and spread via roots and self-seeding. If you cut the plants back after they flower, you'll often receive a second bloom. Keep your arnica healthy by dividing the plants at the roots every 3 years, in either spring or autumn.

# Basil

*Ocimum basilicum*

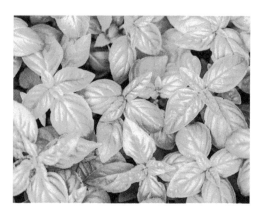

$

Most people are familiar with basil's ability to impart delicious flavor to food; its sweet scent is also unmistakable. But not everyone knows that there are many different varieties of basil, each with antibacterial properties and stomach-settling abilities. A little crushed fresh basil takes the itch out of an insect bite, too.

**Parts Used:** Leaves

**Precautions:** Do not use during pregnancy.

**Identifying/Growing:** You probably won't find basil growing wild, but you can usually find it in the produce department at your local supermarket. Since fresh basil is strongest, and since the plant is very easy to grow, this is one herb that you may want to consider cultivating even if you lack a green thumb.

Basil thrives in the garden or grows just as happily in a pot on a sunny windowsill. It needs lots of light and prefers full sun. It also needs to be watered frequently so the soil stays moist. Harvesting the uppermost leaves will encourage growth and prevent the plant from going to seed.

# Black Cohosh

*Cimicifuga racemosa*

$

*Black cohosh contains isoflavones, compounds that mimic the activity of estrogen. Useful for menopause symptoms, including vaginal dryness, hot flashes, and mild depression, black cohosh also offers anti-inflammatory and pain-relieving benefits. As a cold and flu remedy, it helps quiet coughs while easing discomfort.*

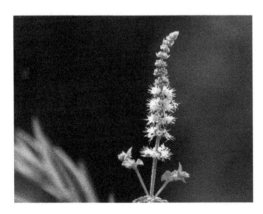

**Parts Used:** Root

**Precautions:** Do not use during pregnancy or breastfeeding. Black cohosh causes gastric discomfort in some individuals; stop using it if this occurs.

**Identifying/Growing:** Black cohosh is indigenous to the eastern half of North America, preferring the edges of fields and open woodlands. With oval-shaped leaves, erect stems that grow to 3 feet or taller, and white flowers on slender spikes, it gets its name from the blackish color of its rootstock.

Black cohosh seeds should be planted in indoor containers in fall and kept in a warm, dry place, preferably one that receives full sunlight. When the plants emerge, water them weekly and keep them indoors until the danger of frost is over. Transplant your black cohosh to a location that receives morning sun but offers afternoon shade. Fertilize the area with well-rotted compost before transplanting and repeat each spring. Water the plants three times per week during dry weather, or even more frequently if you notice that they are beginning to wilt.

# Blue Vervain

*Verbena hastata, Verbena officinalis*

*Blue vervain relaxes the nervous system and offers reliable pain relief, especially when it is used in poultices for rheumatism, joint pain, and neuralgia. In tea, the leaves help ease headache, bladder discomfort, and sore throat. Try blue vervain tea next time you need an expectorant for chest congestion or bronchitis.*

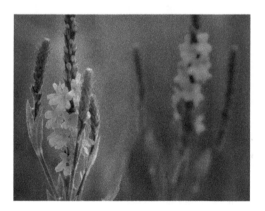

**Parts Used:** Leaves

**Precautions:** Do not use during pregnancy.

**Identifying/Growing:** Blue vervain can be found growing wild in meadows, waste places, and along roadsides through-out most of North America and Europe. Lance-shaped leaves with rough, toothy edges are arranged on stems averaging 3 to 7 feet, and little purplish blue flowers emerge from slender spikes located at the top of the plant.

This lovely herb is easy to grow. Blue vervain needs light to germinate, so simply sow the seeds and water them without covering them with soil. Be sure to keep the seeds moist until they germinate. For stronger remedies, pick the herbs before they flower and dry them right away. Allow some of your blue vervain to flower and go to seed if you'd like a steady supply year after year; it self-seeds and will come back each spring.

# Catnip

*Nepeta cataria*

Ⓢ

*Almost everyone is familiar with catnip, which is an essential treat for our feline friends. Despite its tendency to bring out a cat's playful side, this lovely herb does the opposite in most people, promoting relaxation with none of the unpleasant side effects that accompany pharmaceutical sedatives.*

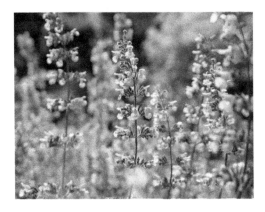

**Parts Used:** Leaves and flowering tops

**Precautions:** Do not use during pregnancy.

**Identifying/Growing:** Catnip can sometimes be found growing wild, usually along roadsides. Its heart-shaped leaves have a soft, minty scent, and are greyish-green with a downy coating. White flowers with lavender-colored spots adorn the upper portion of the plant.

Catnip is a very pretty addition to the garden. Like other members of the mint family, it is easy to grow and has a tendency to spread if you let it. Start the seeds indoors in spring and transplant young seedlings after the danger of frost, placing them in a sunny, well-drained area. Protect your catnip plants from eager felines by covering them with a lid made of chicken wire. You can harvest the leaves and flowers throughout the season, year after year.

# Chamomile

*Matricaria recutita*

$

Gentle yet effective, chamomile offers antibacterial and anti-inflammatory properties. Its ability to soothe the nervous system makes it indispensable in calming and bedtime tea blends, and it offers antispasmodic activity that makes it ideal for treating tense, aching muscles. Next time you are stressed, sore, or sleepless, give chamomile a try.

**Parts Used:** Flowers

**Precautions:** Chamomile contains high levels of coumarin and can adversely interact with blood thinners. It can also cause problems for people who are allergic to ragweed.

**Identifying/Growing:** Chamomile is native to Europe but is very easy to grow in most places. Its small, daisy-like flowers have white petals and raised yellow centers, and its leaves have a fine, feathery appearance. Easy to grow from seed, it makes a beautiful border in the garden and self-seeds year after year. Cut or pick the flowers when they are in full bloom, and expect to enjoy at least two cuttings each summer.

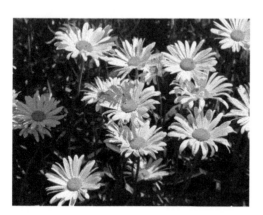

# Chickweed

*Stellaria media*

$

*Chickweed is among the most common wild herbs and can be found growing throughout most of the world. You can use fresh chickweed to make soothing poultices for treating rashes, irritated skin, and minor burns, and the juice helps ease itching. Beyond its usefulness as a medicinal remedy, chickweed makes a tasty addition to spring salads.*

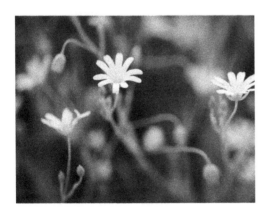

**Parts Used:** Leaves and flowers

**Precautions:** Chickweed can have a laxative effect when eaten in large quantities. Be careful not to wildcraft in areas where fertilizer, pesticide, or herbicide has been applied.

**Identifying/Growing:** You can probably find chickweed growing in your lawn, and it can be found in woods and meadows, too. This hardy little plant grows year-round in many places, fading only when temperatures are below freezing, and quickly reemerging with the slightest hint of warmth. It features tiny white flowers and oval leaves that emerge from low, slender stems averaging 4 to 6 inches long.

Many people try to eradicate chickweed from their lawns, often unsuccessfully. You can encourage it to grow by raking a spot for it, wetting the soil, and spreading the seeds approximately ½ inch apart. Cover the area with a light layer of topsoil, mist it with water, and then leave it undisturbed until the plants establish themselves. Your chickweed will self-seed, and requires nothing in terms of maintenance.

# Comfrey

*Symphytum officinale*

$

Comfrey's Latin name is rooted in the Greek word sympho, *meaning "to make grow together." This refers to its traditional use in speeding the healing of fractures. The plant's ability to alleviate pain and inflammation is also legendary; it works well on cuts, scrapes, insect bites, burns, and rashes, too.*

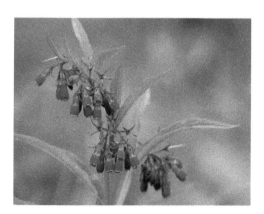

**Parts Used:** Leaves and roots

**Precautions:** Comfrey contains natural insect-repelling pyrrolizidine alkaloids that can be carcinogenic and cause liver damage when the plant is overused internally. Infants and children are most susceptible; use your best judgment when determining whether to take comfrey internally or to reserve it for external use.

**Identifying/Growing:** An herbaceous perennial, comfrey is native to Europe but is easy to grow in partial shade throughout temperate to warm climates. Mature plants attain impressive sizes of 3 to 6 feet high and 2 to 4 feet wide. Comfrey's tiny hanging clusters of pink, violet, or cream-colored flowers rise up from coarse, hairy stems that bear large leaves. The herb is so large that you might think it's a shrub; however, the stems never become woody, and the entire plant dies back in winter.

Comfrey can be grown from seed, but it's far easier to cultivate via root cuttings, which should be planted horizontally at a depth of about 3 inches and spaced approximately 3 feet apart. It thrives in rich, organic soil with plenty of nitrogen. Composting annually will help you get the best possible harvest. You can cut and dry the leaves anytime after the plants reach a height of 2 feet.

# Dandelion

*Taraxacum officinale*

($)

*Dandelion is often thought of as an invasive weed, but its ability to detoxify the liver and help stop indigestion, bloating, and constipation makes it a valuable addition to your garden. While the root offers medicinal properties, the greens make an iron-rich addition to salads, and the fragrant yellow flowers provide pollinators with a good source of nectar.*

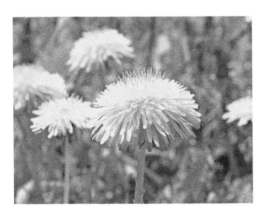

**Parts Used:** Roots and sap

**Precautions:** Dandelions are generally considered safe, but ensure that the ones you harvest have not been exposed to herbicide or pesticide.

**Identifying/Growing:** Long, toothy leaves and fluffy, bright yellow flowers make the dandelion easy to identify. You can encourage dandelions to populate your lawn and garden by skipping herbicides. When harvesting roots and other plant parts, be sure to leave a few plants behind and let them go to seed so that you'll have plenty of dandelions next year.

# Echinacea

*Echinacea angustifolia,*
*Echinacea purpurea,*
*Echinacea pallida*

*Echinacea has a long history of use in wound, infection, and cold care remedies. If you start taking it at the first sign of a cold or the flu, you will find that it reduces the duration and intensity of symptoms, including coughing, fever, and sore throat. Thanks to its antibacterial, antifungal, and antiviral properties, echinacea is useful for treating a variety of ailments.*

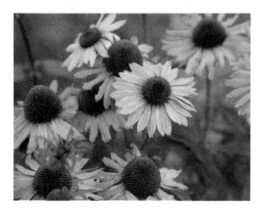

**Parts Used:** Roots

**Precautions:** Echinacea stimulates the immune system and can cause adverse reactions with pharmaceuticals used in immune system suppression therapy. Do not use echinacea if you have a chronic infection such as tuberculosis or HIV/AIDS, or if you have an autoimmune disease such as lupus or rheumatoid arthritis. Echinacea causes allergy symptoms in some people who are allergic to ragweed; stop taking it if it has an adverse effect on you.

**Identifying/Growing:** Also known as purple coneflower, echinacea features vibrant yellow, orange, and red tones in the center of its daisy-like blooms. Although echinacea grows wild in prairies across North America, it has been overharvested and should be cultivated at home rather than wildcrafted.

Echinacea is very easy to grow in your garden, and besides offering wonderful medicinal benefits, it attracts bees and butterflies. This beautiful herb grows to a height of about 4 feet. It will self-sow if allowed to go to seed, and its roots will send up new shoots each year, too. Just provide the plants with a sunny patch of limey, well-drained soil, and it will reward you with beauty and inexpensive remedies.

# Fennel

*Foeniculum vulgare*

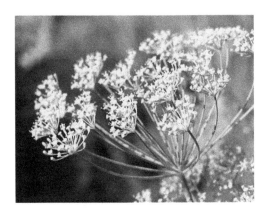

Offering a sweet, licorice-like scent,
fennel is a beloved culinary staple
that is cultivated worldwide. Used
medicinally, its seeds relieve bloating, gas, and abdominal cramps.
Fennel has estrogenic properties
that balance the female reproductive
system, easing menopause and menstrual symptoms.

**Parts Used:** Seeds

**Precautions:** Remedies made with seeds
and other plant parts are generally
considered safe, but you should avoid
fennel essential oil if you are pregnant or
breastfeeding.

**Identifying/Growing:** Feathery, dark-
green leaves and bright green stalks rise
up from fennel's base, which is rounded,
deeply ribbed, and pale greenish-white
in color. The stalks grow to a maximum
height of 5 feet, and the tiny yellow flowers grow in tightly packed groups.

Fennel should be grown in full sun, and
requires a well-drained site. Sow the seeds
12 inches apart and cover them lightly
with about ¼ inch of soil. Water lightly
after seeding, and keep the planting site
moist until shoots appear a week or two
after planting. Prevent toppling by staking
the plants when they reach a height of
18 inches.

Harvest the seeds after they turn brown
but before they start popping off their
umbels on their own. You can make the
process a bit easier by wrapping cheesecloth around the fennel's top and cutting
the stalks. Ensure that the seeds are completely dry before storing them in a tightly
capped jar.

# Feverfew

*Tanacetum parthenium*

$

*Feverfew offers a mild tranquilizing effect that makes it ideal for easing the tension and fatigue that often lead to headaches. It inhibits blood platelets from aggregating in the bloodstream and prevents small capillaries from becoming blocked. This action gives feverfew the ability to prevent and treat migraines.*

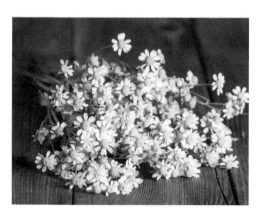

**Parts Used:** Leaves

**Precautions:** Fresh feverfew leaves can cause mouth ulcers. Do not use feverfew during pregnancy and avoid it if you are allergic to ragweed.

**Identifying/Growing:** Feverfew is a close relative of marigolds and dandelions. Its tiny, daisy-like flowers feature cheerful yellow centers and diminutive white petals. It is easy to grow feverfew; simply sow the seeds in a sunny spot during spring or summer. When you harvest the plants, leave some behind and allow them to go to seed so that you'll have a steady supply next year.

# Garlic

*Allium sativum*

$

*Spicy garlic is a culinary staple in many kitchens, but its usefulness extends far beyond its savory flavor. This ubiquitous herb contains over 30 medicinal compounds, including allicin, a broad-spectrum anti-microbial agent. As a medicinal food, it helps prevent blood clotting, lowers triglycerides and cholesterol, and provides essential antioxidants.*

**Parts Used:** Roots

**Precautions:** Overconsumption of garlic can cause gas and heartburn. When used topically, garlic can cause a skin rash in some people with sensitive skin.

**Identifying/Growing:** Garlic is easy to identify and grow, and in many areas you can plant it in fall for a spring harvest, and again in early spring for a second harvest in autumn. Garlic does best in a sunny spot, in soil that has been amended with rich compost. Plant the cloves with their tips up, about 2 inches deep, and then mulch heavily. Allow the soil to dry out between waterings to prevent rotting, and harvest when about half of the leaves turn brown or yellow.

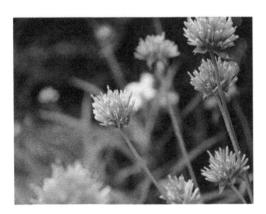

# Ginger

*Zingiber officinale*

( $ )

*A fragrant root that lends itself to use in sweet and savory dishes alike, ginger also proves useful in treating aliments that range from cramps to nausea. It is a natural blood thinner that can lower cholesterol, and its ability to raise body heat and purge toxins makes it ideal for use in cold and flu treatments.*

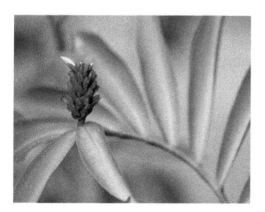

**Parts Used:** Roots

**Precautions:** Because ginger is a blood thinner, you should avoid it if you have a bleeding disorder or gallbladder disease, or if you take prescription blood thinners. Large doses of ginger can stimulate the uterus, so use it cautiously if you are pregnant.

**Identifying/Growing:** Ginger is a tropical plant with waxy leaves and smooth, fragrant white flowers. At the grocer, select roots with a firm feel.

If you live in a tropical climate, you can grow ginger outdoors. In colder areas, you can grow it in a greenhouse or sunny indoor location. Plant the roots in large, wide containers, placing them at a depth of about 10 inches. Ginger plants grow to impressive heights of 4 feet or more, and the blossoms carry a delightful fragrance to reward your effort.

# Ginkgo Biloba

*Ginkgo biloba*

($)

*A beautiful deciduous tree with unique fan-shaped leaves, ginkgo biloba supports healthy circulation while improving cognitive function, maintaining your energy level, and even improving libido in both genders. Ginkgo biloba contains natural antihistamines and anti-inflammatory agents, making it a good choice for treating allergies and asthma naturally.*

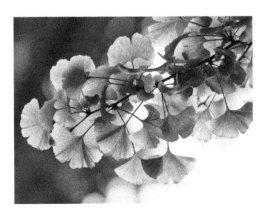

**Parts Used:** Leaves

**Precautions:** Do not take ginkgo biloba if you take prescription monoamine oxidase inhibitor (MAOI) or selective serotonin reuptake inhibitor (SSRI) drugs. Ginkgo enhances the effect of prescription blood thinners; talk with your doctor before using it if you take any of these.

**Identifying/Growing:** Graceful trees with flared, two-lobed leaves, ginkgo biloba can grow to 100 feet tall. Ginkgo trees can live more than 1,000 years, and are immune to disease, insects, and pollution. Beyond their usefulness in herbal medicine, these lovely trees make a stunning addition to your home's landscape. Purchase a sapling from a nursery and put it in a prominent place. Once the tree is mature, you can harvest and use its green leaves anytime from spring to fall.

# Ginseng

*Panax ginseng, Panax quinquefolius*

*Ginseng boosts mood and memory while alleviating the effects of fatigue, stress, and exhaustion. It also enhances your body's immune response, helping to ward off bacteria and viruses. When choosing ginseng, be aware that Siberian ginseng is a separate species with different properties than those offered by Korean and American ginseng.*

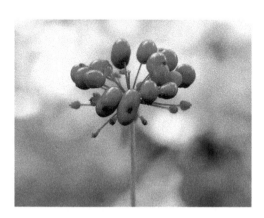

**Parts Used:** Root

**Precautions:** Do not use ginseng during pregnancy. If you have high blood pressure, consult your doctor before using ginseng.

**Identifying/Growing:** A whole ginseng root has an almost human shape, with a forked bottom and sides. Mature plants grow in deciduous forests and are between 10 and 20 inches tall, bearing red berries that drop off to form new plants. If you wildcraft ginseng, be sure to plant these berries.

If you live in a cool, temperate climate and have access to a shady patch of deciduous trees, you may be able to grow ginseng. Begin by having your soil tested. Ginseng grows best at pH levels between 4 and 7. Order ginseng seeds when you have found a suitable site, and plant them according to the accompanying instructions, which should include notes on stratification and sprouting. Your ginseng will take between 4 and 8 years to grow to harvest size.

Be aware that ginseng harvest is tightly regulated in many areas. You may need to obtain a license or permit, so check local regulations before proceeding.

# Goldenseal

*Hydrastis canadensis*

*Thanks to high levels of hydrastine and berberine, goldenseal offers antiviral and antibacterial benefits. A useful herb to keep on hand for general use, goldenseal finds its way into remedies for cuts and wounds, sinus infections, respiratory congestion, sore throats, and more.*

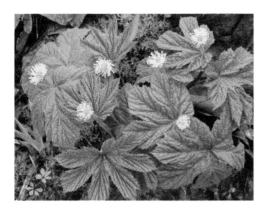

**Parts Used:** Roots, primarily; leaves offer milder benefits

**Precautions:** Do not use goldenseal if you are pregnant or breastfeeding, or if you have high blood pressure. Goldenseal tincture contains concentrated tannins that can cause stomach irritation; stop internal use if this occurs.

**Identifying/Growing:** Wild goldenseal once thrived in shady forests from Minnesota to Georgia, but habitat loss and overharvesting have led to its decline. With leaves and berries resembling those of the raspberry, these perennial shrubs grow to a maximum height of just 10 inches. Roots are thick and knotted, with bright yellow interiors.

You can easily grow goldenseal in a protected area with deep, loamy soil and dappled shade. The rootstock should be divided into sections ½ inch or larger, and should then be placed approximately 8 inches apart at a depth of 2 to 3 inches. Plant the rhizomes in autumn, and keep the area mulched and weeded. Goldenseal has a very slow growth rate and takes up to 2 years to bloom. Your roots should be ready to harvest in 3 to 4 years.

# Hops

*Humulus lupulus*

*If you've ever experienced a slightly sleepy sense of relaxation after drinking a particularly hoppy beer, then you already know a bit about what hops are capable of. Besides acting as a reliable sedative, this herb can ease nervous tension and anxiety, promote healthy digestion, and relieve bladder pain. In menopause, hops can alleviate symptoms such as hot flashes.*

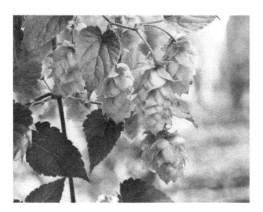

**Parts Used:** Flowers

**Precautions:** Because hops contain a potent plant estrogen called 8-prenylnaringenin, they should not be given to prepubescent children of either gender. Hops are also dangerous for dogs.

**Identifying/Growing:** Hops grow on long vines called bines, which can grow to a length of more than 25 feet. Rarely found in the wild, these lush green plants are typically cultivated by commercial hops growers, who rely on stout trellises to support the bines and keep them well aerated. The medicinal portion of hops is the female flower, which is pale green, with a cone-like shape.

If you have a sunny spot and vertical space for a stout trellis that can support at least 25 pounds, then you may be able to cultivate hops at home. You'll need to grow at least two varieties to allow for cross-pollination, so plan accordingly. Plant the rhizomes in spring, after all danger of frost. Water them frequently and harvest the hops when the cones are filled with a thick, golden powder.

# Horseradish

*Armoracia rusticana*

$

*Offering the ability to clear blocked sinuses, pungent horseradish is more often considered as a condiment than as a medicine. This spicy herb loosens chest congestion, too, and promotes circulation. Horseradish is a useful diuretic that can help you release excess water weight and ease urinary tract infections.*

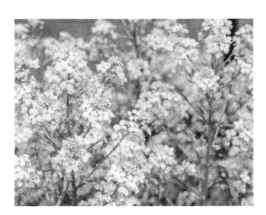

**Parts Used:** Root

**Precautions:** Do not use horseradish if you have low thyroid function, or if you take thyroxine. Topically, overuse may cause blistered skin; discontinue if this occurs. Wildcraft carefully, avoiding areas that have been exposed to herbicides and pesticides.

**Identifying/Growing:** Horseradish has long, compact leaves with a strongly marked central vein. Small white flowers emerge from the stalk in summer. You can find horseradish growing wild in fields, along forest edges, around old homesteads, and in many other places. Just pick a leaf and smell it; if it carries the scent of prepared horseradish, then you know you've struck medicinal gold.

Horseradish is very easy to grow in most climates. It's a good idea to grow your horseradish in containers or select a site away from the rest of your garden plants, as this herb has a habit of taking over. The roots can be dug anytime after the leaves appear.

# Hyssop

*Hyssopus officinalis*

$

*Hyssop is a reliable antiviral and expectorant herb that proves valuable during cold and flu season. Suitable for treating bronchitis and sinus infections too, this sweet-smelling member of the mint family makes a wonderful addition to teas and decoctions.*

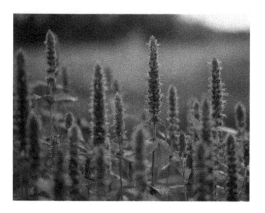

**Parts Used:** Leaves and flowers

**Precautions:** Do not use hyssop if you are pregnant or have epilepsy.

**Identifying/Growing:** This fragrant perennial herb has smooth, narrow leaves and white, pink, or royal blue flowers on tall stalks. It is not often found in the wild but is very easy to grow in most places.

Plant your seeds or seedlings in full sun, and give each one at least 12 inches of space to spread out. Allow the soil to dry out between waterings, and treat the plants to a side dressing of compost each fall. Snip the leaves and blossoms as needed. If you want more hyssop to grow, you can allow it to self-seed, or you can collect the seed capsules after they have dried on top of the plants.

# Licorice

*Glycyrrhiza glabra*

$ $ $

*The roots of the licorice plant are long, fleshy, and sweet. Used for food and medicine by Native Americans, this herb proves useful in treatments for asthma, cold and flu symptoms, and earache. If you have a toothache, you can try chewing on licorice root to ease the pain while you wait for a dental appointment.*

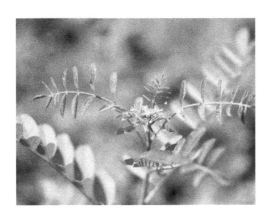

**Parts Used:** Root

**Precautions:** Licorice root is best used in moderation, as overuse can lead to water retention, low potassium, and elevated blood pressure. Do not use licorice root if you have diabetes, heart disease, kidney disease, or hypertension.

**Identifying/Growing:** Licorice has naturalized throughout Asia, Europe, the Mediterranean region, and North America. The plants have light, spreading foliage with small leaflets and graceful flowers in violet, pale blue, pale yellow, or purplish colors. The seeds grow in pods that look like miniature peapods, and the roots penetrate to depths of 3 to 4 feet below the earth's surface.

Start licorice seeds indoors at least 2 weeks before the last frost or plant them in your garden after all danger of frost. Each plant needs at least 36 inches of space to thrive, and needs to be meticulously weeded. The plants may die back during winter but will reemerge in spring. You can dig the roots after 3 to 4 years have passed.

# Milk Thistle

*Silybum marianum*

$

Milk thistle is such a potent detox-ifier that it has gained popularity even outside herbal medicine circles. It contains high levels of silymarin, which helps regenerate damaged liver cells while providing protection from viruses and toxins. If you drink alcohol frequently or take harsh drugs, consider adding milk thistle to your daily regimen.

**Parts Used:** Seeds

**Precautions:** Overuse can lead to mild diarrhea

**Identifying/Growing:** Milk thistles grow to 7 feet tall. Their large, shiny white-veined leaves make them easy to distinguish from other thistle cultivars, but their purple flowers have a similar appearance.

You can easily grow milk thistle in most climates. Direct seed in early spring or late summer, keep the site watered, and allow the plants to grow. Harvest the seed heads when the flowers fade, before the wind carries the seeds away.

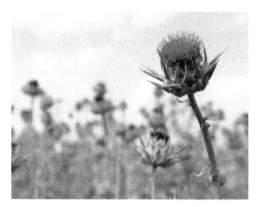

# Mullein

*Verbascum thapsus*

$

*Coughs, earaches, and sore throats are no match for mullein, which offers both analgesic and anti-bacterial properties. A fresh poultice made with ground or mashed mullein leaves makes a good first aid treatment for minor wounds, burns, and insect bites.*

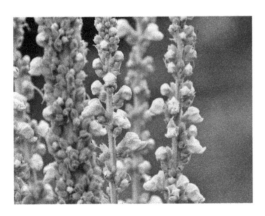

**Parts Used:** Leaves and flowers

**Precautions:** Mullein is generally considered safe. Wildcraft only in areas where you're certain that the soil is free from herbicides, pesticides, and other chemicals.

**Identifying/Growing:** With its tall central spike covered in bright yellow flowers, mullein is easy to spot from a distance. These stately plants grow to an average height of 3 to 4 feet, and are common throughout Europe, North America, and the Mediterranean region.

If you want to grow your own safe supply of mullein, you'll find it simple. Collect seeds from plants after the flowers fade. Pat the seeds onto the soil but don't cover them, as they need light to germinate. Water them and transplant them after the first leaves appear. You can start harvesting leaves the first year, and in the second year, the flowering spike will appear. Collect the flowers, leaves, and buds from mature 2-year-old plants, and leave some plants to reseed the following year.

# Passionflower

*Passiflora incarnate*

*Often used in conjunction with other relaxing herbs like valerian and catnip, passionflower is a mild sedative that can help you fall asleep when your mind is busier than you'd like it to be. As a nerve tonic, passionflower eases anxiety and nervous stress, and can help with nerve pain associated with shingles and neuralgia.*

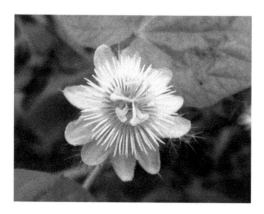

**Parts Used:** Stems and leaves

**Precautions:** Because passionflower can cause uterine contractions, it should not be used during pregnancy. Passionflower can increase testosterone and intensify conditions such as baldness and prostate problems when taken in excess.

**Identifying/Growing:** Passionflower is a vigorous climbing vine with exotic purple blossoms. Native to Central America and Mexico, it is also found growing wild in some parts of the southern United States.

Passionflower can be cultivated as a perennial. You can try to grow this plant from seed, but it is difficult to germinate. The easiest way to propagate passionflower is by taking tip cuttings early in summer. Treat the cuttings with liquid rooting hormone and keep them warm and moist until new growth appears, usually within 2 weeks. Provide a trellis for the passionflower to climb up, and harvest leaves and stems in mid- to late summer.

# Peppermint

*Mentha piperita*

$

*Candy, soap, toothpaste, and other common products often get their flavors and aromas from peppermint. This popular herb is an excellent one for digestive complaints, and it offers relief from body aches, congestion, headaches, and nausea.*

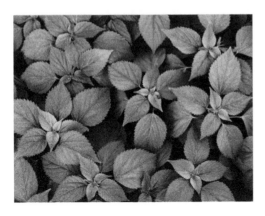

**Parts Used:** Leaves

**Precautions:** Peppermint can aggravate heartburn. Discontinue use if your digestive problems worsen.

**Identifying/Growing:** The easiest way to identify peppermint is by its unmistakable scent. Fresh and crisp, it often greets you before you spot the herbs growing. Peppermint can be wildcrafted in many places; look for it near springs, creeks, and ponds.

You can easily grow peppermint in a pot on your windowsill, or you can enjoy a larger harvest by cultivating some in your garden. Consider dedicating a container to peppermint, as it spreads quickly and can take over more space than you'd like it to if left unchecked. Just plant the seeds in spring, water them, and start harvesting leaves as they mature.

# Plantain

*Plantago major*

$

*An herb so common that it is usually considered to be a weed, the humble plantain offers astringent, antimicrobial, antihistamine, and anti-inflammatory benefits, among many others. All 200 or so plantain species offer similar benefits, and all have been used to treat wounds, insect bites, and other minor ailments since ancient times.*

**Parts Used:** Leaves

**Precautions:** Plantain is generally considered safe. Be sure to wildcraft only in areas where no herbicide, pesticide, or chemical runoff is present.

**Identifying/Growing:** Plantain has elongated oval leaves with well-defined ribs. At maturity, slender spikes emerge from the tops of the plants and bear tiny flowers, often in shades of white or yellow.

If you can't find plantain growing wild, you can order seeds online and plant them in fall or spring in an area with moist soil. Treat your plantain to plenty of water and feed it well with organic compost, and you'll be rewarded with large plants that provide plenty of natural medicine. Once plantain takes root in your garden, it should return year after year.

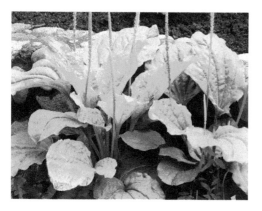

# Raspberry

*Rubus idaeus, Rubus strigosus*

$

Raspberries make a delicious addition to a healthy, natural diet, but don't overlook the leaves when you next harvest these tasty little fruits. Raspberry leaf is an effective, safe remedy for cold and flu symptoms. It also has a long, successful history of being used in teas for relieving menstrual discomfort. As a uterine tonic, raspberry tea can be enjoyed throughout pregnancy.

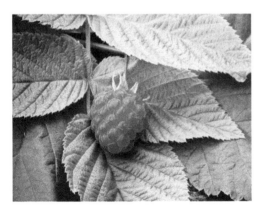

**Parts Used:** Leaves

**Precautions:** Although raspberry leaf is safe for the entire family to use, green leaves can cause nausea. Ensure that raspberry leaves are completely dried before use.

**Identifying/Growing:** With their thorny canes and toothed, deeply ridged leaves, raspberry and black raspberry plants grow wild in many places throughout the world. White, purple, or pink flowers give way to hard green berries that ripen into delicious purple or ruby-red morsels. Whatever variety you wildcraft or cultivate, all offer similar medicinal properties.

You can obtain raspberry bushes from your local nursery and plant them in a sunny spot in your garden or yard. Cover them with a protective net to keep the birds from eating your berries, and harvest the leaves as they mature.

# Rosemary

*Rosmarinus officinalis*

$

*A fragrant herb that's more often thought of as a culinary staple than a medicine, rosemary proves valuable during cold season, when it can be employed in soothing soups and teas that help ease sinus pain. Rosemary stimulates circulation and acts as a tonic for the central nervous system. Its scent improves memory and concentration while providing a quick mood boost.*

**Parts Used:** Leaves

**Precautions:** Do not use if you are pregnant or if you have epilepsy. Although some calming oils like jasmine, ylang-ylang, chamomile, and lavender have been shown to prevent seizures, more pungent oils like rosemary, fennel, sage, eucalyptus, hyssop, camphor, and spike lavender have been known to trigger epileptic incidents.

**Identifying/Growing:** Rosemary is a compact shrub with fragrant, elongated leaves and strong, woody stems. Tiny flowers in shades from white to lavender emerge in late summer.

While it's not likely that you'll find rosemary growing wild, this herb is simple to grow in a warm, sunny spot. Seeds take a long time to mature, so you may find it more convenient to purchase plants from a local nursery. Harvest the leaves early in the morning for stronger flavor and greater efficacy.

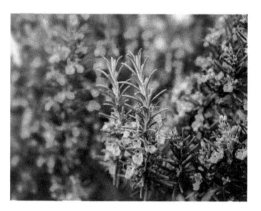

# Sage

*Salvia officinalis*

$

*Although sage is common and inexpensive, it is an excellent remedy for a number of ailments including colds and fevers, hot flashes, painful or heavy periods, rashes, and sore throats. You can even put it to work on painful gums and gingivitis. Try it in culinary applications, where it offers a wonderful taste while helping you heal naturally.*

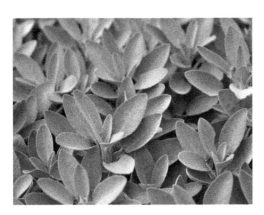

**Parts Used:** Leaves

**Precautions:** Sage is generally considered safe.

**Identifying/Growing:** There are about 900 different *Salvia* species, with some being purely ornamental and others being useful for culinary and medicinal applications. Elongated, soft leaves of silver-green grow on most varieties, along with pinkish to purplish flowers. The stems tend to be woody and erect, and the aroma is fresh, slightly pungent, and a bit mouthwatering.

Sage takes a long time to mature when it is grown from seed, but you can find mature plants at most nurseries and transplant them in a sunny spot. Most sage varieties prefer slightly dry soil; check your plants' requirements for best results.

# Saw Palmetto

*Serenoa serrulata*

ⓢ

*Saw palmetto is best known as an effective herbal remedy for benign prostate hyperplasia, often working faster than prescribed drugs. While it isn't widely recognized by the mainstream medical establishment in the United States, it is widely prescribed throughout Europe.*

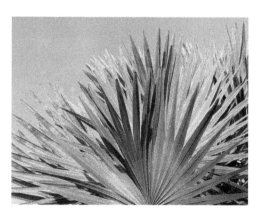

**Parts Used:** Berries

**Precautions:** Saw palmetto is sometimes useful for stopping hair loss in men, but because it increases testosterone, it can cause women to grown unwanted facial hair. If you have acne, saw palmetto may make the condition worse.

**Identifying/Growing:** Saw palmetto is native to the US East Coast and can be found from Florida to South Carolina. The trees are short and scrubby, growing no taller than about 10 feet. Fans of spiky leaves give way to oblong berries, which have a reddish-brown color when ripe. The berries should be dried before use in herbal medicines.

# Skullcap

*Scutellaria lateriflora*

$

*Despite its spooky-sounding name, skullcap is a useful healing herb. A mild sedative that offers quick relief from anxiety, nerve pain, and nervous tension, skullcap can also help ease the uneasy feelings that can accompany menopause.*

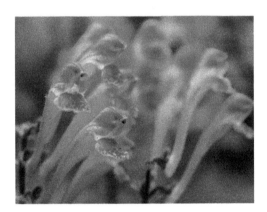

**Parts Used:** Stems, leaves, and flowers

**Precautions:** Do not take skullcap during pregnancy or while breastfeeding. Do not use skullcap if you have liver disease, epilepsy, or a seizure disorder.

**Identifying/Growing:** Skullcap is an herbaceous perennial herb that develops a creeping habit. The flowers are pale to dark blue or purple, with elongated throats and rounded tops that might remind you a bit of snapdragons.

You may be lucky enough to wildcraft skullcap in damp, partly shady areas throughout the United States and Europe, and you can easily grow them in your garden. Begin by refrigerating the seeds for a week, and then plant them in pots or flats. Press the seeds gently to ensure that they have good contact with the soil, and then mist them with water. Cover the container with plastic wrap and place it in a warm, sunny spot such as a windowsill. Remove the plastic wrap when the first green leaves appear, and then mist the little plants lightly each day. Transfer the seedlings to a spot that receives a bit of shade during the summer months and keep them well watered. Harvest the plants as they mature.

# St. John's wort

*Hypericum perforatum*

$

St. John's wort is an effective anti-depressant that can help alleviate anxiety and symptoms associated with mild depression. It is also a strong antiviral herb that can shorten the duration of cold sores when applied topically. Other topical uses include treatment of arthritis, fibromyalgia, muscle aches, and sciatica.

**Parts Used:** Flowers, upper leaves

**Precautions:** Do not take St. John's wort if you take monoamine oxidase inhibitor (MAOI) or selective serotonin reuptake inhibitor (SSRI) medications.

**Identifying/Growing:** The easiest way to take St. John's wort as a dietary supplement is to choose a high-quality standardized product in capsule form and follow recommended dosage instructions. If you'd like to grow your own St. John's wort for use in topical remedies, you'll be rewarded with beautiful, compact plants that yield lots of bright yellow blossoms. It prefers sandy or rocky soil, where it reaches a maximum height of about 2 feet. Once established, St. John's wort requires little care; simply harvest the blooms and upper leaves as they appear.

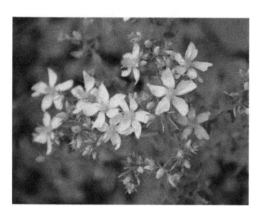

# Thyme

*Thymus vulgaris*

$

*Thanks to its ability to impart a wonderfully savory flavor to foods, thyme is a staple in many kitchens worldwide. This lovely little herb is an excellent overall cold remedy that calms coughing spasms, clears chest congestion, helps you sleep soundly, and soothes sore throats.*

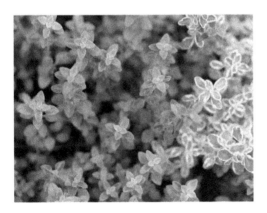

**Parts Used:** Leaves

**Precautions:** Thyme is generally considered safe, but regular overuse can lead to abnormal menstrual cycles.

**Identifying/Growing:** Thyme has an aromatic scent that makes it easy to identify. Tiny oval leaves cling to slender, woody stems, and minuscule pink flowers emerge during spring and summer. There are about 350 variations of this herb, all with slight variations in appearance; however, all offer similar medicinal benefits.

Thyme is simple to grow, particularly if you purchase mature plants and transplant them into a sunny spot. This herb prefers well-drained soil and will creep if not kept contained in a pot. You can begin harvesting the plant tops after the first spring frost, and stop clipping about a month before fall's first frost. Regular harvesting will keep your thyme plants from becoming too woody, and will encourage them to keep on growing tender new leaves for you to enjoy.

# Turmeric

*Curcuma longa*

($)

Turmeric is a fantastic culinary herb with a warm, savory taste. Beyond its usefulness in the kitchen, it contains curcuminoids and curcurmin, which offer excellent anti-inflammatory benefits. Turmeric provides relief from a number of painful conditions including arthritis, rheumatoid arthritis, and psoriasis.

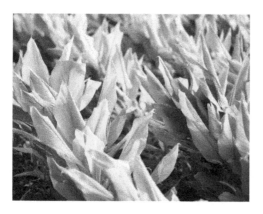

**Parts Used:** Root

**Precautions:** Do not take turmeric in large quantities if you have hypoglycemia. Be careful; the bright yellow color can stain clothing and skin.

**Identifying/Growing:** Turmeric is a tropical plant with large oval-shaped leaves and bright pink flowers. It is native to India but is widely cultivated throughout Bengal, China, and Java. The rhizomes or roots are elongated, and have a bright yellow, orange, or red color.

Because turmeric requires lots of rainfall and warm temperatures to thrive, it is only cultivated in tropical climates. If you can obtain a fresh root, you can try to grow a plant indoors; however, you must keep it well watered and ensure that the temperature never falls below 65 degrees Fahrenheit. It takes approximately 10 months to a year for a new root crop to emerge.

# Valerian

*Valeriana officinalis*

*Best-known as a natural sleep aid, valerian can be used alongside other remedies, especially when pain is preventing you from getting the rest you need. While it is potent and has been compared to valium, it is non-habit-forming. Because it relaxes smooth muscles, valerian is also useful for menstrual cramps.*

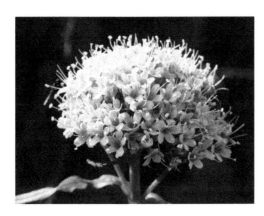

**Parts Used:** Roots

**Precautions:** Valerian is generally considered safe, but it can act as a stimulant in certain individuals. See how this herb affects you before relying on it for relief from insomnia.

**Identifying/Growing:** There are several different valerian cultivars, or varieties, all with similar medicinal effects. The plants feature fern-like leaves and small clusters of white to pink flowers. Capable of growing to heights of 5 feet, these attractive plants add beauty to your garden while providing an ample harvest of natural medicine.

To grow valerian, sow the seeds into warm soil after all danger of frost has passed. Keep your young seedlings watered, and you'll be rewarded with beautiful plants that emit a fragrance that might remind you of vanilla and cinnamon. Harvest the roots in autumn.

# Witch Hazel

*Hamamelis virginiana*

$ $

*Witch hazel is a mild, effective remedy for acne, cuts and scrapes, insect bites, minor burns, and sunburn. It is suitable for all skin types, and offers an astringent property that makes it useful for shrinking swollen veins.*

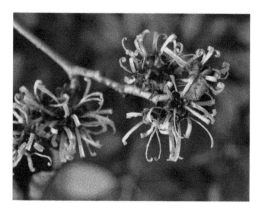

**Parts Used:** Twigs

**Precautions:** Witch hazel is generally considered safe.

**Identifying/Growing:** The easiest way to get your hands on witch hazel is to head to the drugstore, where you'll find the liquid extract alongside other skin care products. If you want to make your own witch hazel extract, you'll need access to witch hazel trees, which grow in the understory of hardwood forests and produce bright yellow blooms in winter after the leaves have fallen off. The leaves are toothed ovals with deeply pronounced veins. Harvest the twigs right after the trees blossom to obtain the strongest extract possible.

# Yarrow

*Achillea millefolium*

$

*Offering a strong medicinal fragrance and fast action, yarrow is a natural styptic, a substance that stops bleeding by contracting body tissue and healing injured blood vessels. Nicknamed the "nosebleed plant," it encourages clotting and helps disinfect minor wounds. When consumed in tea or taken as tincture, it can also help reduce heavy menstrual bleeding.*

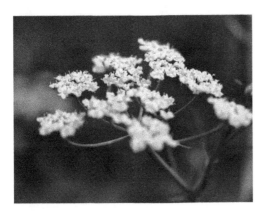

**Parts Used:** Leaves and flowers

**Precautions:** Do not take yarrow internally during pregnancy. Yarrow can cause a rash in some people who are allergic to plants in the Asteraceae family; discontinue use if irritation occurs.

**Identifying/Growing:** Yarrow has soft, feathery, silver-green leaves and tightly packed florets atop strong stems. Most wild yarrow has white or pinkish flowers, but some domestic varieties have yellow or bright pink blooms. This herb grows profusely across North America, Europe, and Asia.

You can very easily grow yarrow in your garden. Simply sow the seeds and keep them watered. Fragrant clusters of leaves will soon be followed by attractive flowers. You can begin harvesting this herb as soon as the plants mature, picking the leaves and flowers in early morning and drying them right away. Since yarrow is a self-seeding perennial, you should only have to plant it once to receive an abundant harvest year after year.

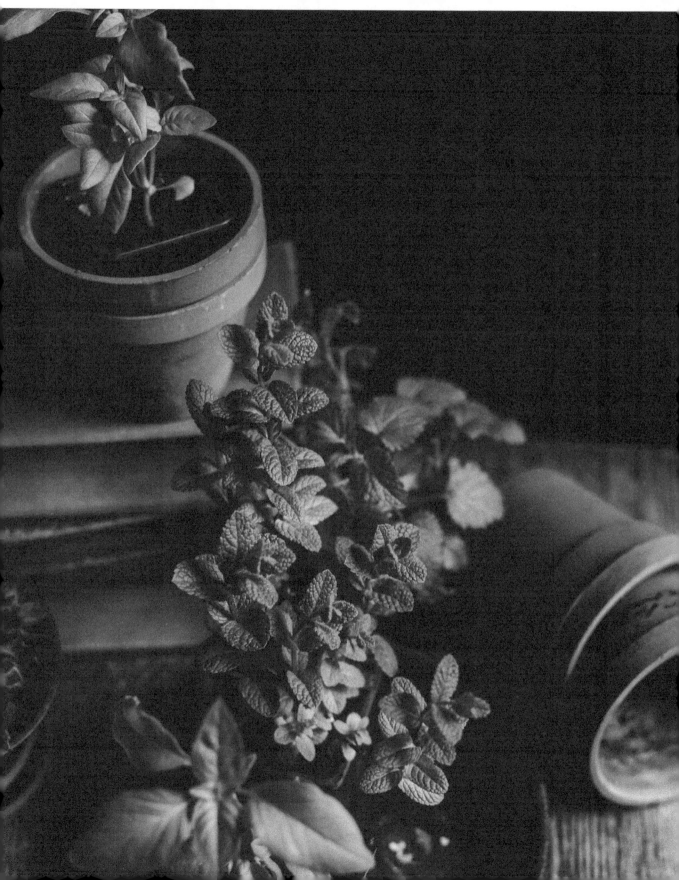

# Appendix

| MEASUREMENT | | CONVERSION |
|---|---|---|
| 1 tablespoon | = | 3 teaspoons |
| 2 tablespoons | = | 1 ounce |
| 4 tablespoons | = | ¼ cup |
| 8 tablespoons | = | ½ cup |
| 12 tablespoons | = | ¾ cup |
| 8 ounces | = | 1 cup |
| 2 cups | = | 1 pint |
| 2 pints | = | 1 quart |
| 4 quarts | = | 1 gallon |

# Glossary

**Analgesic** – A substance that provides pain relief by acting on the central nervous symptom or offering local numbing

**Antibacterial** – A substance that prevents or destroys bacteria, or that slows its multiplication

**Antidepressant** – A substance that can counteract mild depression symptoms

**Antifungal** – A substance that can slow or halt fungal growth

**Antihistamine** – A substance that counteracts the body's response to allergens by opposing histamine receptor activity

**Anti-inflammatory** – A substance that alleviates or prevents inflammation

**Antimicrobial** – A substance that reduces or stops microbial activity

**Antiseptic** – A substance that slows or stops infections

**Antiviral** – A substance that prevents or destroys viruses, or that slows their replication

**Astringent** – A substance that reduces swelling and inflammation by prompting tissue to contract or tighten

**Diuretic** – A substance that stimulates urine production and removes excess water from body tissues

**Expectorant** – A substance that helps expel mucus and phlegm from the lungs by stimulating a productive cough

**Febrifuge** – A substance that reduces body temperature to alleviate fever

**Laxative** – A substance that promotes bowel movements

**Sedative** – A substance that promotes calming, relaxation, or sleep

**Styptic** – A substance that slows or stops minor bleeding

# Resources

## Popular Brands

When you start shopping for convenient herbal remedies, such as premade tinctures and capsules, you'll notice that there are many brands available. Here is a short list of some of the most popular, reliable ones. Conduct research before purchasing supplements from a brand you don't recognize, and be suspicious if prices for prepared products seem too low. Unscrupulous manufacturers often cut corners and use fillers.

- Carlson Labs
- Dr. Mercola
- Gaia Herbs
- Herb Pharm
- Irwin Naturals
- Kirkland
- Mountain Rose Herbs
- Natrol
- Nature Made
- New Chapter
- Nordic Naturals
- NOW Foods
- Puritan's Pride
- Rainbow Light Nutritional Systems
- Schiff
- Trader Darwin's

## Books

Visit your local bookstore or library, and you'll probably find plenty of informative books that can help you deepen your knowledge of herbal medicine. Here are five to consider:

- *The Complete Medicinal Herbal* by Penelope Ody
- *Prescription for Herbal Healing* by Phyllis A. Balch and Stacy Bell
- *Encyclopedia of Herbal Medicine* by Andrew Chevallier
- *The Herbal Apothecary* by J. J. Pursell
- *Rosemary Gladstar's Medicinal Herbs* by Rosemary Gladstar

# Websites

You can find many excellent sources for bulk herbs and supplies online. Here is a list of some of the most popular, best-stocked sites.

- Bulk Apothecary
  www.bulkapothecary.com
- Jean's Greens
  www.jeansgreens.com
- Living Earth Herbs
  www.livingearthherbs.com
- Mountain Rose Herbs
  www.mountainroseherbs.com
- Pacific Botanicals
  www.pacificbotanicals.com
- Starwest Botanicals
  www.starwest-botanicals.com

# Continuing Education

There are many ways to expand your knowledge of medicinal herbs and their uses for natural healing. For example, you can probably find a local wildcrafting class by conducting a quick online search.

If formal education is your goal, then you can seek out a local herbal medicine program to gain a wealth of practical information by learning in person. In the event that you don't have access to an herbal medicine program, or would prefer to take online courses or conduct your own research, you'll find this list of resources helpful.

- **HerbMed**—This electronic database includes a public site with evidence-based information about 20 of the most common herbs. A subscription to HerbMed Pro provides access to a database of information on 255 herbs. You can choose an inexpensive pay-per-day option if you prefer. www.herbmed.org

- **National Center for Complementary and Integrative Health: Herbs at a Glance**—An extensive site with free downloadable fact sheets and an ebook, this resource provides common names, scientific information, precautions, and additional resources for learning about more than 50 popular herbs. www.nccih.nih.gov/health/herbsataglance.htm

- **American Herbalists Guild**—This site provides an impressive menu of offerings. Free professional herbalist training webinars are a good place to begin. www.americanherbalistsguild.com

- **Learning Herbs**—This user-friendly site provides an ample amount of free information, plus some paid content including HerbMentor, a community filled with articles, herbalism courses, reference materials, video tutorials, and more. www.learningherbs.com

- **Vermont Center for Integrative Herbalism**—Classes, training programs, and a library of resources, including informative articles, are just some of the offerings you'll find here. www.vtherbcenter.org/resources/publicationsmedia

# Ailments and Remedies
## Quick Reference Guide

| AILMENT | SUGGESTED HERBS | METHODS OF APPLICATION |
|---|---|---|
| Abscess | Echinacea, goldenseal, yarrow | Topical |
| Acne | Agrimony, aloe, calendula, chamomile, comfrey, sage | Topical |
| Allergies | Feverfew, garlic, gingko biloba, peppermint | Ingestion |
| Asthma | Garlic, gingko biloba, peppermint, rosemary, thyme | Ingestion, inhalation |
| Athlete's foot | Garlic, goldenseal | Topical |
| Backache | Blue vervain, ginger, passionflower, peppermint | Ingestion, topical |
| Bee sting | Aloe, comfrey, echinacea, plantain | Topical |
| Bloating | Dandelion, fennel, peppermint | Ingestion |
| Bronchitis | Garlic, goldenseal, hyssop, licorice, peppermint, rosemary | Ingestion, Inhalation |
| Bruise | Arnica, comfrey, hyssop, witch hazel | Topical |
| Burn | Aloe, chickweed, comfrey, hyssop, mullein, plantain | Topical |
| Canker sore | Calendula, goldenseal | Topical |
| Chapped lips | Aloe, calendula, comfrey, hyssop | Topical |
| Chest congestion | Angelica, goldenseal, hyssop, sage | Ingestion, inhalation |
| Chicken pox | Aloe, calendula, comfrey, echinacea, goldenseal, licorice | Topical |
| Cold | Comfrey, echinacea, garlic, ginger, horseradish, licorice, mullein, raspberry leaf, sage, thyme | Ingestion, inhalation |
| Cold sore | Echinacea, garlic, sage, goldenseal, St. John's wort | Topical, ingestion |
| Colic | Chamomile, fennel, ginger, peppermint | Ingestion |
| Conjunctivitis | Calendula, chamomile, goldenseal | Topical |
| Constipation | Aloe, chickweed, dandelion | Ingestion |

| AILMENT | SUGGESTED HERBS | METHODS OF APPLICATION |
|---------|-----------------|------------------------|
| Cough | Fennel, hyssop, licorice, mullein, sage, thyme | Ingestion |
| Cuts and scrapes | Aloe, calendula, chamomile, comfrey, goldenseal, plantain, thyme | Topical |
| Dandruff | Echinacea, rosemary | Topical |
| Diaper rash | Aloe, chamomile, comfrey, echinacea, thyme | Topical |
| Diarrhea | Agrimony, catnip, goldenseal, raspberry leaf | Ingestion |
| Dry skin | Aloe, calendula, chickweed, comfrey | Topical |
| Earache | Blue vervain, chamomile, echinacea, garlic, goldenseal, mullein | Topical, ingestion |
| Eczema | Aloe, calendula, chamomile, comfrey, goldenseal | Topical |
| Fatigue | Feverfew, licorice, rosemary | Ingestion |
| Fever | Blue vervain, feverfew, raspberry leaf | Ingestion |
| Flatulence | Angelica, fennel, ginger, peppermint | Ingestion |
| Flu | Catnip, chamomile, echinacea, garlic, goldenseal, hyssop, St. John's wort | Ingestion |
| Gingivitis | Calendula, chamomile, goldenseal, sage | Topical |
| Hair loss | Ginger, ginkgo biloba, rosemary | Topical, ingestion |
| Halitosis | Fennel, ginger, peppermint, sage | Topical |
| Hangover | Feverfew, hops, milk thistle | Ingestion |
| Headache | Blue vervain, catnip, feverfew, skullcap | Ingestion |
| Heartburn | Angelica, fennel, ginger | Ingestion |
| Hemorrhoids | Aloe, calendula, chickweed, comfrey, goldenseal, St. John's wort, witch hazel | Topical |
| High blood pressure | Angelica, dandelion, lavender, rosemary | Ingestion |
| Hives | Chamomile, comfrey, licorice, rosemary | Topical |
| Indigestion | Angelica, chamomile, fennel, ginger, peppermint, rosemary | Ingestion |
| Insect bites | Basil, comfrey, echinacea, mullein, peppermint, plantain | Topical |
| Insomnia | Catnip, chamomile, hops, passionflower, valerian | Ingestion |
| Jock itch | Calendula, chamomile, garlic, goldenseal | Topical |
| Keratosis pilaris | Aloe, calendula, chamomile, chickweed | Topical |
| Laryngitis | Ginger, licorice, mullein, sage | Ingestion |
| Menopause | Black cohosh, fennel, sage | Ingestion |

| AILMENT | SUGGESTED HERBS | METHODS OF APPLICATION |
|---|---|---|
| Mental focus | Basil, ginkgo biloba, ginseng, rosemary, sage | Ingestion, inhalation |
| Mental wellness | Angelica, basil, chamomile, ginseng, hops, hyssop, licorice, passionflower, skullcap, St. John's wort | Ingestion |
| Muscle cramps | Ginger, rosemary | Topical |
| Nausea | Chamomile, ginger, peppermint, raspberry leaf | Ingestion |
| Oily skin | Peppermint, rosemary, witch hazel | Topical |
| Poison ivy | Calendula, chamomile, chickweed, comfrey, licorice | Topical |
| Premenstrual syndrome (PMS) | Black cohosh, dandelion, ginger, St. John's wort, raspberry leaf, rosemary | Ingestion |
| Prostatitis | Hops, saw palmetto, turmeric | Ingestion |
| Psoriasis | Chamomile, comfrey, goldenseal, licorice | Topical |
| Rheumatoid arthritis | Blue vervain, comfrey, ginger, licorice, rosemary | Topical |
| Ringworm | Garlic, goldenseal | Topical |
| Rosacea | Aloe, chamomile, feverfew, licorice | Topical |
| Shingles | Comfrey, goldenseal, licorice | Topical |
| Sinus infection | Echinacea, goldenseal, horseradish, hyssop, peppermint | Ingestion, inhalation |
| Skin tag | Dandelion, garlic, ginger | Topical |
| Sore muscles | Fennel, ginger, hops, peppermint, St. John's wort | Topical |
| Sore throat | Agrimony, comfrey, licorice, peppermint, sage | Topical, ingestion |
| Sprain | Arnica, comfrey, ginger, peppermint, rosemary | Topical |
| Stiff joints | Comfrey, ginger, horseradish, peppermint | Topical |
| Sunburn | Aloe, comfrey, hyssop, witch hazel | Topical |
| Tendinitis | Ginger, peppermint, turmeric | Topical |
| Travel sickness | Chamomile, ginger | Ingestion |
| Urinary tract infection (UTI) | Dandelion, horseradish | Ingestion |
| Warts | Basil, garlic, horseradish | Topical |
| Weight loss | Chickweed, dandelion, fennel, ginseng | Ingestion |
| Wrinkles | Aloe, calendula | Topical |
| Yeast infection | Calendula, chamomile, echinacea, garlic, passionflower | Topical |

# References

American Society for Pharmacology and Experimental Therapeutics. "Metabolism of 8-Prenylynaringenin, a Potent Phytoestrogen from Hops *(Humulus lupulus)*, by Human Liver Mircrosomes." Accessed September 14, 2016. dmd.aspetjournals.org /content/32/2/272.full.

Balch, Phyllis A., and Stacy Bell. *Prescription for Herbal Healing,* 2nd ed. New York: Avery, 2012.

Chevallier, Andrew. *Encyclopedia of Herbal Medicine.* New York: Dorling Kindersley, 2000.

Chevallier, Andrew. *Visual Reference Guides Herbal Remedies.* New York: Metro Books, 2016.

Gladstar, Rosemary. *Rosemary Gladstar's Herbal Recipes for Vibrant Health.* North Adams, MA: Storey, 2008.

Gladstar, Rosemary. *Rosemary Gladstar's Medicinal Herbs.* North Adams, MA: Storey, 2012.

Green, James. *The Herbal Medicine-Maker's Handbook: A Home Manual.* New York: Crossing Press, 2002.

Hudson, Tori. "Hops and Menopausal Symptoms," Dr. Tori Hudson. October 12, 2010. www.drtorihudson.com/menopause /hops-and-menopausal-symptoms.

Medicine Hunter. "Medicinal Plants." Accessed September 16, 2016. www.medicinehunter.com /medicinal-plants.

Ody, Penelope. *The Complete Medicinal Herbal.* New York: Dorling Kindersley, 1993.

Pursell, J. J. *The Herbal Apothecary.* Portland, OR: Timber Press, 2015.

Tourles, Stephanie L. *Hands-On Healing Remedies.* North Adams, MA: Storey, 2012.

Weil, Andrew. *Natural Health, Natural Medicine.* New York: Houghton Mifflin, 2004.

Wood, Matthew. *The Earthwise Herbal.* Berkeley, CA: North Atlantic Books, 2008.

# Recipe Index

# General Index